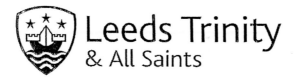

Leeds Trinity
& All Saints

e and Science

Psychology

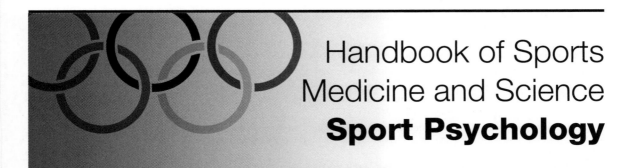

Handbook of Sports Medicine and Science
Sport Psychology

EDITED BY

Britton W. Brewer PhD

Department of Psychology
Springfield College
Springfield, MA
USA

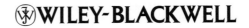

A John Wiley & Sons, Ltd., Publication

This edition first published 2009, © 2009 by International Olympic Committee
Published by Blackwell Publishing

Blackwell Publishing was acquired by John Wiley & Sons in February 2007. Blackwell's publishing program has been merged with Wiley's global Scientific, Technical and Medical business to form Wiley-Blackwell.

Registered office: John Wiley & Sons Ltd, The Atrium, Southern Gate, Chichester, West Sussex, PO19 8SQ, UK

Editorial offices: 9600 Garsington Road, Oxford, OX4 2DQ, UK
                The Atrium, Southern Gate, Chichester, West Sussex, PO19 8SQ, UK
                111 River Street, Hoboken, NJ 07030-5774, USA

For details of our global editorial offices, for customer services and for information about how to apply for permission to reuse the copyright material in this book please see our website at www.wiley.com/wiley-blackwell

Library of Congress Cataloging-in-Publication Data

Sport psychology / edited by Britton W. Brewer.
       p. cm.—(Handbook of sports medicine and science)
    Includes bibliographical references and index.
    ISBN 978-1-4051-7363-6 (alk. paper)
    1. Sports—Psychological aspects—Handbooks, manuals, etc. I. Brewer, Britton W. II. IOC Medical Commmission. Sub-Commission on Publications in the Sport Sciences. III. Series.
    [DNLM: 1. Sports—psychology. 2. Adaptation, Psychological. 3. Stress, Psychological—psychology. QT 260 S7516 2009]
    GV706.4.S677 2009
    796.01—dc22

                                                        2008039505

ISBN: 978-1-4051-7363-6

A catalogue record for this book is available from the British Library.

Set in 8.75/12 pt ITC Stone Serif Medium by Charon Tec Ltd (A Macmillan Company), Chennai, India (www.macmillansolutions.com)

Printed and bound in Malaysia by KHL Printing Co Sdn Bhd.
1—2009

Contents

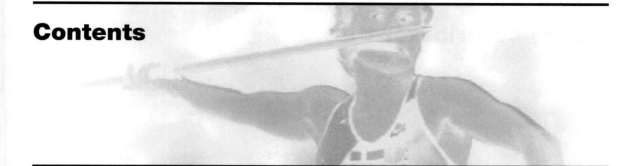

List of contributors

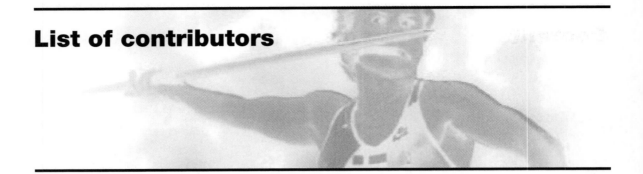

Mark B. Andersen, Ph.D.
School of Human Movement, Recreation, and
Performance and the Centre for Ageing, Rehabilitation,
Exercise, and Sport, Victoria University, Melbourne,
Australia

Eric Bean, M.S.
Department of Kinesiology, Institute for the Study of
Youth Sports, Michigan State University, East Lansing,
MI, USA

Britton W. Brewer, Ph.D.
Department of Psychology, Springfield College,
Springfield, MA, USA

Shauna M. Burke, Ph.D.
Bachelor of Health Sciences Program, University of
Western Ontario, London, Ontario, Canada

Albert V. Carron, Ph.D.
School of Kinesiology, University of Western Ontario,
London, Ontario, Canada

M. Ryan Flett, M.Sci.
Department of Kinesiology, Institute for the Study of
Youth Sports, Michigan State University, East Lansing,
MI, USA

Daniel Gould, Ph.D.
Department of Kinesiology, Institute for the Study of
Youth Sports, Michigan State University, East Lansing,
MI, USA

Sheldon Hanton, Ph.D.
Cardiff School of Sport, University of Wales Institute,
Cardiff, United Kingdom

Nicole M. LaVoi, Ph.D.
Tucker Center for Research on Girls & Women in
Sport, School of Kinesiology, University of Minnesota,
Minneapolis, MN, USA

Stephen D. Mellalieu
Department of Sports Science, Swansea University,
Swansea, United Kingdom

Aidan P. Moran, Ph.D.
School of Psychology, University College, Dublin,
National University of Ireland, Ireland

Jens Omli, Ph.D.
Tucker Center for Research on Girls & Women in
Sport, School of Kinesiology, University of Minnesota,
Minneapolis, MN, USA

Albert J. Petitpas, Ed.D.
Department of Psychology, Springfield College,
Springfield, MA, USA

Kim M. Shapcott
School of Kinesiology, University of Western Ontario,
London, Ontario, Canada

Owen Thomas, Ph.D.
Cardiff School of Sport, University of Wales Institute,
Cardiff, United Kingdom

Robin S. Vealey, Ph.D.
Department of Kinesiology and Health, Miami
University, Oxford, OH, USA

Robert S. Weinberg, Ph.D.
Department of Kinesiology and Health, Miami
University, Oxford, OH, USA

Diane M. Wiese-Bjornstal, Ph.D.
Tucker Center for Research on Girls & Women in
Sport, School of Kinesiology, University of Minnesota,
Minneapolis, MN, USA

Foreword

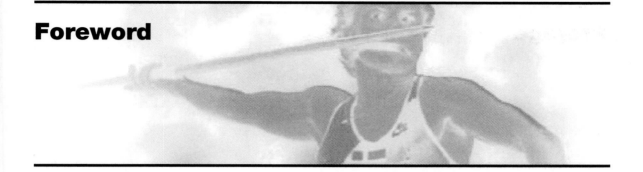

The previous volumes of the Handbooks of Sports Medicine and Science have dealt in comprehensive fashion with Olympic sports in terms of the physical, biomechanical, physiological, and clinical aspects of conditioning and competition. A wide variety of topics have been included as related to the physiological requirements of the various sports and events, conditioning for competition, sports nutrition, as well as injury prevention, treatment, and rehabilitation. Throughout each volume, there has been frequent mention of the involvement of psychology, but no in-depth discussions have been included.

As it was considered to be of great importance to present a comprehensive review of the area of sport psychology in the Handbook series, the Medical Commission embarked on a project to produce this volume, a landmark publication in the areas of sports medicine and the sports sciences. The Editor and the Contributing Authors for this Handbook are to be congratulated on their comprehensive examination of all aspects of the psychological aspects of performance in Olympic sports.

We welcome the Handbook on Sport Psychology to the series of Handbooks of Sports Medicine and Science. Prof. Britton C. Brewer and the contributors have produced a work of excellence that will serve as a valued reference by medical doctors, allied health personnel, coaches, and athletes for many years to come.

Jacques Rogge

Preface

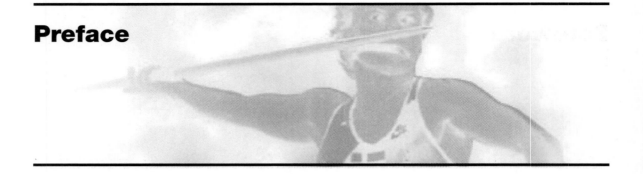

Sport history is replete with examples of athletes and teams that appear to have had a knack for coming through when the pressure is on and conquering the competition despite the obstacles and distractions they encountered in their quest for excellence. Athletes and teams of this sort are often described as having a "mental edge" over the opposition. There are also vivid cases in which unheralded athletes and teams have upset their more highly touted opponents to emerge triumphant in major competitions. Although some unexpected successes can be attributed to physical factors, environmental influences, and just plain bad luck on the part of the vanquished athletes and teams, other instances can be credited to the influence of psychological factors. It is these psychological influences on sport performance that constitute the primary focus of this handbook.

Sport performance has been the subject of psychological inquiry for more than a century, and a concise summary of what is known about the effects of motivation, cognition, stress, confidence, mental preparation, and team dynamics on performance is presented in the current volume. Empirically-validated psychological interventions designed to enhance sport performance are identified and illustrated in case study material at the end of each chapter. Reflecting the breadth of contemporary sport psychology, a substantial portion of the handbook is devoted to psychological research and practice in areas not explicitly pertaining to performance, such as injury, psychopathology, child and adolescent development, and sport career termination. Exploration of such issues underscores the emphasis of the discipline on the well-being of athletes both on and off the field of play.

Completing a project of the magnitude of this handbook would not have been possible without the stellar contributions of many people. The International Olympic Committee Medical Commission supported the project and entrusted me with the responsibility of bringing it to fruition. Howard Knuttgen, Ph.D. nurtured the handbook from its inception and provided sage guidance and vital assistance throughout the publication process. Developmental editors Adam Gilbert, Julie Elliott, Victoria Pittman, and, especially, Cathryn Gates of Wiley-Blackwell kept the project on task and, along with project manager Geetha Williams, helped turn the manuscript into the polished product held by readers. The distinguished and dedicated corps of chapter authors from around the world sacrificed many hours to share their expertise. To these individuals and to others closely involved in producing the handbook, I extend my heartfelt appreciation and gratitude.

Britton W. Brewer, 2008

Chapter 1
Introduction

Britton W. Brewer

Department of Psychology, Springfield College, Springfield, MA, USA

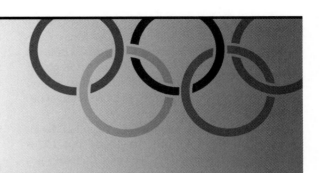

Sport is generally considered a primarily physical endeavor, involving the marshaling of bodily resources to complete a variety of specialized, demanding physical tasks. Undeniably, physical attributes such as speed, strength, stamina, fitness, coordination, agility, flexibility, and resilience are richly rewarded in competitive sport. Recognizing the abundant physical component of sport performance, scientists have investigated biomechanical, physiological, nutritional, metabolic, epidemiological, biochemical, pharmacological, and medical aspects of sport. Applied practitioners in exercise physiology, physiotherapy, sport biomechanics, sports medicine, sports nutrition, strength and conditioning, and other disciplines have translated research findings into interventions designed to enhance the physical performance capabilities of the athletes.

Despite the pronounced emphasis on physical matters in the sport sciences, it is widely accepted that sport performance is influenced not only by physical attributes, but also by psychological factors. Some athletes seem to have a mental edge over other athletes with comparable physical characteristics and training backgrounds. Some athletes perform better under pressure, implement strategies more effectively, tolerate discomfort better, concentrate more intensely, identify more creative solutions to challenging sport situations, push

themselves harder, learn new skills more quickly, or prepare themselves for competition better than their physically similar peers. Issues associated with the mental advantage gained by these athletes fall squarely within the domain of sport psychology. If psychology is the scientific study of behavior and mental processes, then sport psychology is the scientific study of behavior and mental processes *in the context of sport*. Paralleling the rise of other sport sciences, a large research literature has accumulated to inform the practice of coaches and sport psychology specialists. The purpose of this chapter is to present an introduction to sport psychology. Following a brief summary of the historical underpinnings of the field, the current status of sport psychology is reviewed.

Historical underpinnings

The use of psychological methods to calm the mind, relax the body, or otherwise alter mental and physical states of being dates back millennia, particularly in several Eastern traditions. The use of such methods for the enhancement of sport performance is, however, a more recent phenomenon. Shortly after the emergence of psychology as a science in the late nineteenth century, researchers turned their attention to psychological influences on sport behavior. Among the early studies in the annals of psychology is Triplett's famous experiment on the effects of the presence of a fellow competitor on bicycling performance. Recognizing the potential

Sport Psychology. 1st edition. Edited by Britton Brewer.
Published 2009 by Blackwell Publishing.
ISBN 978-1-4051-7363-6.

for application of psychological principles to the realm of sport performance, the Chicago Cubs baseball team hired Coleman Griffith, a scholar at the University of Illinois, as a sport psychologist in the 1920s. Several decades later, the Soviet Union employed sport psychologists as assistant coaches on national teams.

Despite these early scientific and applied developments, it was not until the 1960s and 1970s that sport psychology crystallized as a discipline and forged a distinct identity. Sport psychology textbooks were published and professional organizations such as the International Society of Sport Psychology, the North American Society for the Psychology of Sport and Physical Activity, and the Fédération Européenne de Psychologie des Sports et des Activité Corporelles were founded in the 1960s. Scholarly journals devoted specifically to sport psychology, such as the *International Journal of Sport Psychology*, the *Journal of Sport Behavior*, and the *Journal of Sport Psychology* (later the *Journal of Sport and Exercise Psychology*), appeared in the 1970s. The field expanded further in the 1980s and 1990s as specialized academic training programs in sport psychology mushroomed around the world and criteria for certification as a sport psychology practitioner were established in Australia, the United Kingdom, and the United States.

Current status

Sport psychology has matured to the point that competitive athletes are generally aware of the existence of sport psychologists, although they may not fully know what sport psychologists *do* and how they do it. Sport psychologists work with a variety of client types on a variety of issues using a variety of methods. Despite this variety, some trends have emerged in the work of sport psychologists.

Sport psychology clients

Typically, athletes who consult sport psychologists are competitive, participating at the elite, professional, or university level. Young athletes, masters athletes, and adult recreational athletes may also enlist the services of a sport psychologist. It is common for sport psychologists to consult with coaches, offering information, and working collaboratively to address the psychological needs of athletes on the team. Less frequently, sport psychologists may consult with sport administrators and sports medicine professionals to deal with issues of a psychological nature at the organizational or individual level.

Sport psychology issues

Many of the issues for which sport psychologists are consulted are performance-related. Issues pertaining to motivation, focus/concentration, thought patterns, arousal control, confidence, and mental preparation are common performance-related reasons for seeking the services of a sport psychologist. Because motivation is central to so many aspects of sport involvement—from choosing to participate in the first place and dedicating oneself to extensive training regimens to persisting despite obstacles and exerting effort in the face of discomfort—it is not surprising that many people associate sport psychology primarily with motivation. Sport psychologists work with individual athletes to help them identify appropriate sources and achieve desired levels of motivation for practice and competition. Coaches and administrators may enlist the services of sport psychologists to assist in establishing a sport environment with a motivational climate that is conducive to optimal team functioning.

In most sports, performance can be adversely affected when the attention of athletes is not focused appropriately on the sport task. Athletes who have trouble concentrating or who are distracted by intrusive thoughts are likely to encounter performance difficulties. Sport psychologists can assist athletes in directing their attention to cues that can facilitate enhanced performance.

Sport performance is often impaired when athletes experience levels of arousal or anxiety that are incongruent with their personal preferences or the demands of the sport in which they participate. For example, performance on tasks such as shooting a rifle or attempting a free throw in basketball can be hampered by excessive levels of anxiety and the psychological as well as physiological effects that they have on athletes. Similarly, the performance of athletes who are not sufficiently energized before or during competition may also suffer. In these circumstances, sport psychologists work with athletes helping them to cope with the stressful situations they inevitably encounter in competitive sport and to identify and achieve levels of arousal that are optimal for their sport tasks.

One of the factors that commonly accompanies and indeed may precipitate anxiety in athletes is a lack of confidence. When athletes doubt themselves or believe themselves incapable of completing various sport tasks, their performance may suffer and their confidence may spiral further downward. Sport psychologists can intervene to help bolster the confidence of athletes and set the stage for enhanced performance.

Athletes spend hundreds of hours preparing themselves physically for competition. Some athletes squander their extensive physical preparation by failing to prepare themselves mentally for competition. Other athletes, however, complement their physical training with mental training that prepares them maximally for the wide range of circumstances they may face before and during the competition. Sport psychologists can facilitate mental preparation by helping athletes to anticipate likely and unlikely-but-possible competition-day events and to develop routines as well as plans to deal with such events.

Having a sport team filled with highly talented individual superstar athletes is a desirable situation, but is no guarantee of sport success. Sport history is replete with examples of seemingly undertalented squads that have excelled in the competitive arena. What accounts for discrepancies of this sort? Overachieving teams are often described as having "chemistry" or cohesion that enables them to overcome the odds and achieve success against more talented teams. Sport psychologists work with groups and teams to help them function more effectively as a unit and, ultimately, perform better.

In addition to performance-related concerns, some of the issues for which sport psychologists are consulted have broader implications than purely those for sport performance. Although injuries, for example, can be clearly detrimental to the performance of athletes, they can also have ramifications for long-term physical functioning. In keeping with this broader focus, sport psychologists can help

athletes prevent, adjust to, or recover from injury. Similarly, depending on their educational background, they can help athletes deal with personal problems that affect their lives off the field or help to diagnose behavioral problems (such as eating disorders or substance abuse) that can influence sport performance. Further, because athletes often begin their involvement in sport early in the lifespan, sport psychologists can help coaches and parents to ensure that young athletes are brought along in environments that are conducive to positive physical and psychological development. At the other end of the developmental spectrum, because athletes are frequently involved in competitive sport for a limited period of time, sport psychologists can also assist athletes in preparing for their lives and careers after their playing days are done.

Sport psychology methods

Sport psychologists use a variety of methods to help athletes address their concerns, with the specific techniques and approach depending on the nature of the problem and the resources as well as the preferences of the athlete. Several techniques, however, are used frequently across multiple types of problems for which sport psychologists are consulted, especially those that are performance-related. These techniques, which are often combined in the form of *psychological skills training*, are goal setting, relaxation, imagery, and self-talk.

In goal setting, it is typical for athletes and sport psychologists (and sometimes coaches) to collaborate in establishing a set of behavioral targets that the athletes then attempt to achieve. Generally, sport psychologists encourage athletes to set goals that correspond to specific, measurable behaviors (such as practicing a sport skill a certain number of times on a given day). These are phrased in positive terms (as behaviors to achieve rather than behaviors avoid), and are challenging yet realistic. Although athletes readily set goals referring to sport outcomes (such as victories in particular competitions), outcomes are often beyond their control. Athletes may be able to control their own fitness, preparation, and effort in competition, but they often cannot control the opposition and environmental conditions that can have a large impact on the sport outcomes they ultimately incur. Consequently, goal setting principles commonly refer to the need to set goals for both individually controllable processes as well as sport outcomes, under which athletes have less complete control but which may have greater inspirational value. To maximize the impact of goal setting, sport psychologists generally recommend that athletes record their goals in written form and lay them out on a timetable, from short term to long term. By charting their progress toward goal achievement on a regular basis, athletes can readily evaluate the effectiveness of the goal setting intervention and determine whether they need to adjust their goals—upward or downward—to ensure that the goals are both challenging and attainable. Further, by learning to identify potential barriers to goal attainment and develop strategies to get around such roadblocks, athletes can arm themselves with a means of persisting and continuing to pursue their important aspirations in the face of adversity.

Relaxation training involves teaching athletes to voluntarily decrease the amount of tension in their muscles, calm their minds, and decrease autonomic responses such as their heart rate and blood pressure. In one common method known as progressive relaxation training, athletes are instructed to alternately tense and relax various muscle groups in an attempt to discern the difference between tension and relaxation, and, ultimately, gain the capability of relaxing their muscles at will. In another common form of relaxation training, athletes are asked to engage in various breathing exercises that induce a relaxation response through the taking of deep, diaphragmatic breaths. In autogenic training, a third relaxation training method, athletes learn to relax their bodies by giving themselves suggestions regarding their breathing rate and the temperature as well as heaviness of various parts of the body. With sufficient practice, athletes can use self-instructions such as "my left arm is warm" and "my arms and legs are heavy" to achieve a state of relaxation on a consistent basis.

Imagery is a versatile technique in which athletes are guided to create mental images in which multiple senses are engaged. Sometimes paired with relaxation training, imagery can be used for assisting in the acquisition of a new physical or mental skill, rehearsing a previously acquired physical or mental skill, learning a new strategy, and many other functions in sport psychology. The content of the images varies according to the reason the technique is being used. For example, when imagery is used to foster the development of a physical skill such as a golf swing, sport psychologists are likely to instruct athletes to use visual, auditory, kinesthetic, and other sorts of images that correspond to swinging a golf club. Some imagery instructions involve adopting an internal perspective, in which the athletes are asked to imagine particular settings or situations as experienced through their own senses. Viewing a scene through one's own eyes, as cyclists might view the roadway ahead of them, would be an example of internal imagery. Imagery from an external perspective, in contrast, involves athletes viewing themselves performing specific actions as other people would see them, as if they had been filmed and were watching themselves on a video monitor.

Self-talk, which refers to one's internal dialog with oneself, can be used to influence how athletes think, feel, and behave. For example, negative self-talk, which includes pessimistic, critical statements about oneself and one's prospects for the future, is considered especially detrimental to sport outcomes. Consequently, sport psychologists generally encourage athletes to use self-talk that is positive, which can instill a sense of optimism, or instructional, which directs athletes toward the task at hand. Implementation of a self-talk training program is often preceded by an assessment of athletes' typical self-talk patterns—both what they say to themselves and the circumstances under which they say it—and identification of any irrational or unusual beliefs or expectations that might underlie the athletes' counterproductive thoughts.

Although presented separately, the four methods (i.e., goal setting, relaxation training, imagery, and self-talk) are readily integrated within a single psychological skills training program when appropriate. Moreover, the methods are complementary. For example, relaxation training can be used to produce a calm state that is conducive to generating mental images. Similarly, athletes can use self-talk to trigger mental images that help themselves achieve a more relaxed state. Athletes who are disinclined to implement relaxation, imagery, or self-talk into their training program can use goal setting to enhance their adherence to the program.

In addition to these well-known methods, sport psychologists use a variety of other techniques to address the concerns of athletes. Among the factors that influence the specific approach to assessment and intervention taken by sport psychologists in working with athletes are the characteristics of the athletes' focal problems, the nature of the education and training of the sport psychologists, and the strengths, weaknesses, and preferences of the athletes. A skier with pre-race jitters would almost certainly be treated with different methods than a figure skater with an eating disorder. An athlete with a strong visual sense might display a preference for imagery-based approaches, whereas an athlete who thinks readily in terms of words might elect a program involving modification of self-talk.

Applied issues

Sport psychologists are confronted with several challenging issues that pertain to professional practice with client populations. As an interdisciplinary field, sport psychology has benefited richly from the input from professionals in physical education, psychology, and the sport and exercise sciences. Because sport psychology is simultaneously a subfield of psychology and one of the sport and exercise sciences, there has been controversy on the appropriate education, training, and credentials required for sport psychologists. This controversy has translated into confusion for prospective students in sport psychology and for coaches, athletes, and administrators who wish to receive sport psychology services. Recent credentialing and certification efforts, such as those by the Association for Applied Sport Psychology, the Australian Psychological Society's College of Sport Psychologists, and the British Association of Sport and Exercise Sciences, have eased the confusion, but public awareness of these programs is not yet sufficient to enable consumers to identify appropriately qualified practitioners on a global basis. Unfortunately, practitioners without appropriate training and experience in sport psychology

sometimes attract clients who lack the pertinent information needed to evaluate the qualifications of prospective consultants.

As a subfield of psychology, sport psychology is guided by a code of ethics. Among the ethical issues that are particularly salient in sport psychology are competence, confidentiality, and multiple relationships. As in many other professions, sport psychologists are ethically bound not to offer services for which they are not sufficiently competent to provide. Given that trust is the pillar on which relationships between athletes and sport psychologists rests and that matters of a personal and private nature are often discussed in consulting sessions, it is not surprising that confidentiality is paramount in applied sport psychology. It is essential for sport psychologists not to share information about their clients with others unless they have received written consent from their clients to do so. Even in situations where coaches or team administrators are paying for the sport psychology services, it is inappropriate for sport psychologists to share information without the athlete's consent. Another aspect of ethical behavior in sport psychology that can cause misunderstanding if not clarified at the outset of the consulting relationship is the prohibition on avoidable multiple relationships. Sport psychologists should not, for example, simultaneously serve as an athlete's sport psychology consultant and fellow nightclub attendee.

Conclusions

Sport psychology has emerged as a field with a research tradition that provides a foundation for direct application with athletes. As the role played by psychological factors in the performance and overall well-being of athletes has become better understood, interventions have been designed to favorably affect athlete behavior throughout their involvement in sport and beyond. Although practiced widely among elite athletes in many sports, sport psychology is still gaining acceptance. With further expansion of the field comes the potential to help ensure that the psychological needs of athletes at all levels of competition are addressed.

Further reading

Hanton, S., Mellalieu, S. (eds.) (2006) *Literature Reviews in Sport Psychology*. Nova, New York.

Moran, A.P. (2004) *Sport Psychology: A Critical Introduction*. Routledge, New York.

Tenenbaum, G., Eklund, R.E. (eds.) (2007) *Handbook of Sport Psychology*, 3rd Edn. Wiley, New York.

Weinberg, R.S., Gould, D. (2006) *Foundations of Sport and Exercise Psychology*, 4th Edn. Human Kinetics, Champaign.

Williams, J.M. (ed.) (2006) *Applied Sport Psychology: Personal Growth to Peak Performance* 5th Edn. McGraw-Hill, Boston.

Chapter 2
Motivation

Robert S. Weinberg

Department of Kinesiology and Health, Miami University, Oxford, OH, USA

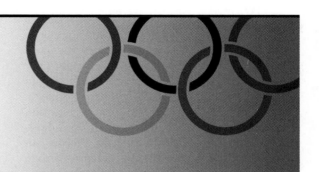

Introduction

One of the most consistent characteristics of great coaches, teachers, and leaders is that they are all great motivators. Specifically, they can get individuals to perform up to their various levels of ability as well as get them to work together for the betterment of the team/group. Similarly, great performers are highly motivated to hone their skills, practicing consistently for many years to reach their goals. Thus, the motivation to practice, condition, and persevere, with the commitment to improve and attain a level of excellence, is at the heart of achieving. The coaches, teachers, and performers who have been successful over time have learned the value of inspiration, perspiration, and dedication. In essence, motivation, whether it's internal or external, or whether it involves motivating oneself or others, is a key determinant in reaching one's potential in sport.

Along these lines, it is important to understand what are the most effective methods of motivation (both those that are both more extrinsic and more intrinsic). In either case, the focus is usually to enhance persistence, intensity, effort, drive, and determination. In fact, research has revealed that motivation can influence the selection of an activity, continuing involvement (persistence), effort in practice and competition, and quality of performance.

Sport Psychology. 1st edition. Edited by Britton Brewer.
Published 2009 by Blackwell Publishing.
ISBN 978-1-4051-7363-6.

It would be impossible to review and discuss all the different motivational approaches and techniques that are used in sport and physical activity. Therefore, this chapter focuses on those approaches and techniques that have received consistent empirical support in the literature. In addition, in discussing these, only the key points are highlighted because it is beyond the scope of the chapter to discuss the techniques in great detail and depth. Finally, clear practical information is presented so that coaches and athletes can readily translate them according to their own specific situation. Thus, the different topics that are addressed include: (a) goal setting, (b) goal orientation, (c) rewards/punishments, and (d) intrinsic motivation. Before addressing these topics, a brief overview of the concept of motivation is warranted.

Defining motivation

Motivation can simply be defined as the direction and intensity of one's effort. The direction of effort refers to whether an individual seeks out approaches or is attracted to certain situations. For example, a college student might be motivated to join an athletics club, a coach might choose to attend a coaching clinic, or an athlete may seek out a rehabilitation professional to receive treatment for an injury. Intensity of effort refers to how much effort a person puts forth in a particular situation. For instance, a volleyball player may attend practices (approach) but not put forth a lot of effort during these practices. Conversely, a gymnast may want to score high on a routine to help her team so badly that she becomes over motivated and performs poorly. Finally, a weight lifter may train 6 days a week like his teammates, but put forth more effort and intensity into each workout.

Although it is convenient to separate direction from intensity of effort, for most people direction and intensity of effort are closely related. In most cases, if a basketball player always arrives early to practice, he is probably going to expend a great deal of energy and effort during the practice. Conversely, if a player typically comes late to practice and misses several practices, he would likely not exert great effort at practice.

Interactional approach

One of the key tenets to understanding people in general and motivation in particular is that both individuals and situations must be understood to provide for optimal motivation. More specifically, both individual factors such as personality, needs, goals, and interests and situational factors such as coaching/teaching style, win–loss record, support of the community, and tradition as well as how individual and situational factors interact need to be considered when trying to determine the most effective way to motivate. Although one might have a general principle that says positive reinforcement is the best way to motivate athletes, punishment might indeed be more effective for a specific athlete (e.g., one who is very competitive) in a specific situation (e.g., when at the end of close, important games). In essence, there is a science and an art of coaching and teaching. Scientists attempt to find general principles that apply to most people in most situations, but good coaches and teachers know when to apply these principles and to whom, which is the art of coaching and teaching.

Strategies to enhance motivation

The focus of this chapter is on general principles and theories of motivation to enhance performance

and well-being. As noted earlier, it is the job of coaches and athletes to apply these principles in their specific situations. Many coaches say that motivating athletes is their primary responsibility after teaching them the basic skills of the sport. But it's the ability of the coach to motivate athletes to learn the skills and techniques and then to apply them to competitive situations that is critical. Some of the most studied and effective motivational strategies used by coaches are discussed as follows.

Goal setting

One of the most robust findings in the scientific literature is the effect of goal setting on task performance. There have been many reviews of literature on the effectiveness of goal setting in industry and sport. Both the literatures indicate that setting goals can significantly enhance performance. In fact, a survey of leading sport psychology consultants working with Olympic athletes in the United States revealed that goal setting was the most frequently used psychological intervention in both individual and group consultations. But the important point is that goal setting will not automatically improve performance. Rather, one has to set the proper types of goals to make them most effective.

Before discussing specific principles, a general point should be made regarding the differences among outcome, performance, and process goals. Outcome goals are the most popular and usually are concerned with winning and losing, such as having a goal to win a tournament or place first in a swim meet. There is nothing wrong with setting an outcome goal. The problem is that too many performers focus too much on this outcome and thus put pressure on themselves. In addition, outcome goals are not under a person's control and thus one might, for example, swim a personal best, but still come in fourth place because the other swimmers were better and also swam extremely well. Performance goals focus on the actual performance such as running the 1500m in 4:50 or shooting 80% from the foul line in basketball. There is no mention of the outcome and thus the performance is solely or predominantly under one's own control. Finally, there are process goals, which focus mostly on the process of reaching one's performance goals. For example, process goals might be getting one's racquet back early in tennis right after the opponent strikes the ball, or extending one's arms when swinging a bat in baseball. Research and practice have revealed that performance and process goals should be emphasized and outcome goals minimized. In essence, reaching one's process and performance goals increase the likelihood of achieving one's outcome goals.

There are four primary reasons why goals work:

1. Goals direct attention to important elements of the skill being performed. Research with athletes has confirmed that the primary reason performers set goals is to provide direction and focus to their actions.

2. Goals mobilize performer efforts. Athletes often get discouraged in their attempts to reach certain levels of performance due to obstacles such as injury. Setting a series of short-term goals, for example, helps athletes put forth effort to reach these goals.

3. Goals prolong performer's persistence. Following-up on the increased effort noted earlier, goals help performers persist over time as they strive to reach their goals. For example, a person who wants to lose 20 kg might be easily discouraged, as this seems like a lot of weight (and it is) and a very daunting task. But if one can break that down to losing 1 kg a week, it seems more manageable, and motivation and persistence can remain high for a long period of time.

4. Goals foster the development of new learning strategies. For example, if a basketball player's goal is to increase her free-throw percentage from 70% to 80%, she might refine her pre-shot routine, change the biomechanics of her shot, or practice more shots even when she feels tired. These new learning strategies can serve as action plans to help achieve goals.

Although many principles can be gleaned from both the laboratory and the field studies that have been conducted, there are a couple of useful acronyms that incorporate many of these concepts and serve as goal setting guidelines for athletes and coaches. The first is known as SMARTS. In essence, goals should be (a) specific, (b) measurable, (c) action-oriented, (d) realistic, (e) timely, and (f) self-determined. The second acronym is known as INSPIRED. That is, goals should be (a) internalized, (b) nurturing, (c) specific, (d) planned, (e) in your control, (f) reviewed regularly, (g) energizing, and (h) documented. Many of the same principles are seen in both of these acronyms, although there are some differences because all goal setting principles cannot be captured in one simple acronym.

With respect to the specificity and measurability of goals in the SMARTS acronym, goals that are general and difficult to measure (e.g., "I just want to improve my game" or "I want to do my best") do not produce as much performance improvement as goals that are specific and measurable (e.g., "I want to improve my first serve percentage in matches from 55% to 60%"). Providing a specific goal allows athletes to receive feedback on how they are doing in relation to the goal. If, for example, a tennis player's first serve percentage goes down from 55% to 52%, she knows that she is not moving toward her goal. This feedback helps motivation and persistence in providing consistent effort to reach the goal. In addition, it allows the athlete to reevaluate her goal and make it easier (e.g., 57%) or more difficult (e.g., 63%), depending on the feedback that is received.

A critical point is having an action plan to reach one's goal. Too often, athletes set outcome goals such as winning a tournament or conference championship, but there is no real plan regarding what to do to reach this goal. For example, if a runner's goal is to win the 1500 m race in competition a month from now (an outcome goal), what would the runner need to do in order to reach this goal? A better goal (because it would be under the runner's control) would be to reduce one's 1500 m time from 4:45 to 4:40 in the next race. However, it would still be important to set action-oriented goals to help reach this goal. For example, the runner might set goals in terms of the number of 400 m runs performed in practice, the number of times certain lifts are done in the weight room, the kinds of foods eaten, and so forth. These goals would be very specific, but accomplishing them should help the runner reach the goal of running a 4:40 in the next 1500 m race.

Of course, the goal should be realistic—not too easy and not too difficult. In essence, the goal should be difficult to achieve, but attainable with consistent effort. But the "R" could also stand for reevaluating goals and possibly changing them if they prove to be too easy or too difficult. Goals are a starting place, not an ending place. For example, if a baseball player set a goal to bat .300 and at midseason he was hitting .220, then it would seem appropriate to reevaluate the goal and reset it for, maybe, .275.

Goals should be timely in that there should be a time or date by which they should be accomplished. In the goal of running 4:40 for the 1500 m race, there is obviously a time frame because the race is coming up in 1 month. Similarly, if one's goal was to lose 20 kg, a time frame should be set and there should even be some short-term goals with a time frame (e.g., losing 5 kg a month or 1 kg a week). This would add to the specificity of the goal as well as provide feedbacks on how one is doing in trying to reach the goal.

Finally, for maximum commitment, goals should be self-determined.

That is, goals should be set by the athlete (not by the coach, parent, or teammate), although certainly input could be received from these individuals, especially if they have expertise in the area. But the more that goals can be determined and set by the athletes, the more committed they will be and the more persistence they will display in attempting to achieve these goals.

Goal orientation

Closely related to goal setting are the goal orientations inherent in individuals. In recent years, researchers and practitioners have come to understand that success and failure are not concrete events, but instead depend on athletes' perceptions of whether they have reached their personal goals. In essence, whether athletes perceive an outcome as a success or failure depends on how they define success or failure in the first place. This perception will have obvious implications for an athlete's confidence, interest, effort, and persistence in the task.

Research has revealed two predominant goal orientations. Task- (or mastery-) oriented athletes are concerned with development of their competence and ability to improve in a task. They tend to view ability as being determined by their improvement and are satisfied if their performance reflects extracting the best out of their current ability by mastering a particular technique, increasing tactical awareness, or making improvements in learning or performing a task.

In contrast, ego- (or competitive-) oriented athletes view success purely in terms of comparisons with others. The criteria for a high perception of ability and achievement is beating the opposition or achieving a similar result at the expense of observably less effort. In essence, to feel successful and competent, ego-oriented athletes have to demonstrate ability superior to someone else, regardless of personal improvements or developments.

So what are the implications of understanding these two different goal orientations in terms of motivation? Along these lines, factors such as persistence, taking personal responsibility, anxiety, enjoyment, intrinsic motivation, and performance have all been linked to task- and ego-oriented goals. However, it should be noted that task- and ego-oriented goals are independent. Athletes could be high on both, low on both, or high on one and low on the other. Generally speaking, task-oriented goals have been linked to more positive outcomes than ego-oriented goals. Most Olympic athletes are high on both task- and ego-orientation. The trick is to balance task- and ego-orientation in both competing hard and trying to win at the same time.

Highly competitive sport typically emphasizes an ego orientation with a focus on winning. High-level coaches know that their jobs are based on winning, and professional athletes also know that winning brings more publicity and bigger financial contracts. Although an ego orientation might be useful in certain circumstances, athletes and coaches need a complementary task orientation to maximize intrinsic motivation, long-term growth, persistence, and, eventually, performance. Interestingly, research has revealed that the more athletes are solely interested in winning, the less likely they are to win. Although at first glance this seems contradictory, the increased desire to win usually

Table 2.1 Competitive performance mentality.

Helps athletes balance the self-challenge (task goals) versus the game challenge (ego goals) inherent in every competition. After every competition, it is critical to review and appraise the self-challenge first (i.e., level of individual skills and efforts relative to personal expectations) and then review the game challenge by reflecting on the skills of the opponent and aspects that tested the athlete's resources in competition.

Creating an achievement log and answering the following questions can help athletes understand the different types of goals they should set.

Examples of questions relating to a task-oriented focus
Where did I show the most improvement?
When did I work the hardest?
What was the most fun aspect?
Under what conditions did I perform best?

Examples of questions relating to an ego-oriented focus
When was I superior to my opponent?
When was I able to do things others weren't able to do?
What conditions led me to beat others?

results in too much pressure being put on athletes (or they put it on themselves).

Thus, the challenge is to focus on how athletes can develop skills to enhance their task orientation, stimulate task involvement, and manage their ego orientations. One approach, a system called competitive performance mentality (CPM), is essentially a mind-set that reflects both task- and ego-oriented goals, but it does so in a way that doesn't excessively pressure athletes to prove themselves to others (i.e., it reduces social comparison). The CPM (Table 2.1) reflects the way in which athletes deal with the self-challenge and competitive challenge that sport typically provides. Specifically, the self-challenge focuses on athletes striving to perform at their best and thus success is defined (and satisfaction enhanced) in relation to their own level of ability. Although this should be the primary focus, there is also a competitive challenge that focuses on how athletes perceive that they performed in relation to their competition (i.e., winning is the focus). Self- and competitive challenges exist in every competition, and athletes need to try to meet these challenges. Then, athletes should reflect upon and appraise whether the challenges were met successfully and why and how the challenges were or were not accomplished.

As noted earlier, there will almost always be a focus on the competitive challenge from the

media, spectators, friends, family, and society in general. It is the job of athletes in the CPM to be able to focus on the important skills or qualities regarding the self-challenge, as they reflect upon the qualities that are important to personal performance. The competitive challenges should be noted, but not emphasized, as this will be done by others. Although it may be difficult to change an athlete's goal orientation in a short period of time, coaches could change the motivational climate to emphasize individual performance improvements rather than outcomes of competitions.

One thing that athletes can do to promote a task orientation (and focus on self-challenge) is to complete a daily or weekly achievement log. This system encourages athletes to set maintenance or improvement goals (see section on goal setting) as well as record their thoughts and feelings regarding their striving to reach these goals. This system of goal setting helps athletes take greater responsibility for evaluating themselves on controllable behaviors that are critical to their success.

The second thing that athletes can do to promote a task orientation is to set process and performance goals as discussed earlier. These goals can be both for training and competition but the focus is now on what athletes need to do to perform well rather than on the outcome of the event. This focus can be encouraged by coaches by asking questions based on the athlete's own performance. For example, "how well did you play today?" or "how positive were your thoughts throughout the competition?" These types of questions help athletes focus more on their performance than on the outcome of the competition. The task-oriented values of taking personal responsibility, and focusing more on effort and mastery help create a task-oriented motivational climate. Coaches can develop a "language logbook" in which they note times when they have purposely used task-involving comments to help athletes focus on performance and process rather than outcome.

Reinforcement/feedback

Probably the method most often employed by coaches to motivate athletes is the use of some sort of reinforcement and feedback. The theory behind the use of feedback is based on operant conditioning principles, that argue that our behaviors can be influenced by, and eventually controlled by, manipulating consequences. Specifically, if the consequences for a behavior are positive, then this increases the likelihood of performing the behavior. Conversely, if the consequences of a behavior are negative, then the likelihood of performing the behavior is reduced. For example, if a baseball player receives positive feedback from the coach for putting forth full effort, then the athlete is more likely to try hard in the future. However, if the player is yelled at for "slacking off" on a drill, then the athlete is less likely to "slack off" again. Unfortunately, although this approach may generally work, things are not always so simple. For example, some athletes perform better after negative feedback than positive feedback, sometimes athletes actually perceive a punishment as a reward, and, at times, they may be unable to repeat the reinforced behavior.

Positive approach

Research has generally revealed that the positive approach to reinforcement and feedback, which aims at strengthening desired behaviors through the use of encouragement, positive reinforcement, and sound technical instruction carried out within a supportive environment produces the most optimal outcomes. The negative approach, which emphasizes punishment, should only be used occasionally and within the context of the positive approach. When used sparingly, the potential impact of punishment is increased. In essence, the positive approach, through its emphasis on improving rather than on "not screwing up," fosters a more positive learning environment and tends to promote more positive relationships between coaches and athletes.

Types of reinforcers

There are several ways coaches can use positive reinforcement to enhance performance and other positive behaviors.

First, the most effective reinforcer needs to be chosen, a process that requires sensitivity to the needs of individual performers. Potential reinforcers include social behaviors such as verbal praise, non-verbal signs (e.g., applause, smiles), physical contact (e.g., pat on the back), and the opportunity to engage in certain behaviors (e.g., extra batting practice) or play with a particular piece of equipment. Material rewards such as money, medals, varsity jackets, and trophies can also serve as reinforcers. Overall, reinforcers should be varied so a coach does not sound too repetitive. It is important for coaches to get to know athletes' likes and dislikes to help determine the most effective reinforcers for them. Finally, research has revealed that if a verbal reinforcement is combined with specific instructions on the correct way to perform the behavior, the effectiveness of the reinforcer is increased. For example, telling a basketball player "nice shot, I liked the way you followed through" gives the player positive feedback while providing a cue for how to shoot the shot correctly.

Schedules and timing of reinforcement

A frequently asked question is how often and how consistently reinforcement should be given. The most important distinction is between continuous and intermittent reinforcement. Continuous reinforcement means that reinforcement is given every time athletes perform the desired behavior, whereas intermittent reinforcement involves providing reinforcement to athletes only occasionally after they exhibit the desired behavior. In general, when an individual is learning a skill, a continuous schedule is recommended because it not only strengthens the desired response, but also provides the performer with frequent feedback about how he or she is doing. However, once the skill becomes well-learned, an intermittent schedule is more desirable as research has revealed that behaviors reinforced on partial schedules persist much longer in the absence of reinforcement than do those that have been reinforced only on a continuous schedule.

Reward successful approximations

When individuals are acquiring a new skill, especially a complex one, they inevitably make mistakes. It may take weeks and countless trials to master the skill, which can be disappointing and frustrating to the learner. It is helpful, therefore, to reward small improvements that approximate the desired performance as the skill is being learned. This technique, called shaping, allows people to continue to improve as they get closer and closer to the desired response. For example, if players are learning the overhand volleyball serve, they might first be rewarded for performing the proper toss, then the proper motion, then good contact, and finally the execution that puts all the parts together successfully.

Reward emotional and social skills

In today's world of sport, the pressure to win can seep down from the professionals to youth sport participants. However, sport can be a breeding ground to learn a variety of life skills. More specifically, athletes who demonstrate good sporting behavior, responsibility, judgment, and other signs of self-control and cooperation should be recognized and rewarded. This becomes even more important as young athletes look up to sport heroes as role models and, unfortunately, are often disappointed. One of the reasons that National Basketball Association administrators were so dismayed over the 2005 fight between the Detroit Pistons and Indiana Pacers and the fans (which resulted in significant suspensions of several players) was the message it sent to youngsters. Many people believe that learning these life skills is even more important than learning specific sport skills and thus the chance to reward emotional and social skills, especially in younger participants, should not be overlooked.

Reward effort, not only outcome

Once again, with the focus on winning and outcome, the notion of effort, although appreciated, often is not rewarded. The notion of focusing on effort instead of winning is highlighted by the quote from all-time basketball coaching legend, John Wooden (as quoted in Weinberg & Gould, 2007):

> You cannot find a player who ever played for me at UCLA that can tell you he ever heard me mention winning a basketball game. He might say I inferred a little here and there, but I never mentioned winning. Yet the last thing that I told my players, just prior to tip-off, before we would go out on the floor was, when the game is over, I want your head up—and I know of only one way for your head to be up—and that's for you to know you did your best. This means to do the best you can do. That's the best; no one can do more .... You made that effort.

Interestingly, a study with children showed that performers who received effort-oriented feedback ("good try") displayed better performance than those provided ability-oriented feedback ("you're talented"), especially after failure. Specifically, after failure, children who were praised for effort displayed more task persistence, more task enjoyment, and better performance than children praised for high ability. Thus, effort (which is under one's control) appears to be critical to producing persistence, which is one of the most highly valued attributes in the sport environment.

Punishment

Although positive reinforcement should be the predominant way to change behavior (in fact, most researchers would argue that 80%–90% of feedback should be positive), at times punishment is necessary and is often used as a means of controlling behavior. For example, the judicial system predominantly uses punishment when someone breaks the law. The threat of punishment, theoretically, stops many individuals from breaking the law in the first place. When using punishment, there are some guidelines to make it more effective and some recommendations for what *not* to do (see Table 2.2).

Intrinsic motivation

One of the topics that has interested both researchers and practitioners in terms of motivation is the distinction between intrinsic and extrinsic

Table 2.2 Guidelines for using punishment.

- Be consistent by giving everyone the same type of punishment for breaking similar rules.
- Punish the behavior and not the person. Convey to the individual that it's his or her behavior that needs to change.
- Allow participants to have input in making up punishments for breaking rules.
- Do not use physical activity as a punishment.
- Impose punishment impersonally—do not berate athletes or yell. Simply inform them of the punishment.

Things to avoid when using punishment include:
- Intimidation. Don't berate a person in front of the group/team.
- Criticism. Do not criticize during a competition.
- Physical abuse. Never use physical abuse as a punishment (e.g., hitting a player, making players run in hot weather because they did something wrong).
- Guilt. Do not use guilt to make players feel ashamed for what they did (e.g., "they let down the entire team").

---

motivation. Although external rewards can enhance motivation and increase performance, research has revealed that external rewards, under certain conditions, can undermine intrinsic motivation. In addition, intrinsic motivation is often seen as the stronger (or at least longer lasting) type of motivation. In this section, both of these ideas are addressed in focusing on how to enhance motivation, especially from an intrinsic perspective.

What is intrinsic motivation?

Motivation can come not only from external sources, but also from inside the person. Intrinsic motivation focuses on striving inwardly to be competent and self-determining in the quest to master the task at hand. In sport, intrinsically motivated people tend to enjoy competition, like the action and excitement, focus on having fun, and want to learn skills to the best of their ability. The focus is not on financial gain, getting one's name in the newspaper, or some other form of extrinsic achievement or recognition. Rather, it is participating for the pride one gets in performing the activity for itself and the pure love of the activity. For example, Steve Ovett, a former elite middle-distance runner, when asked why he ran competitively, responded, 'I just did it because I wanted to … to get the best out of myself for all the effort

I'd put in." (Hemery, as cited in Weinberg & Gould, 2007) Interestingly, a study investigating the sustained motivation of elite athletes found that the athletes were driven mostly by personal goals, rather than financial incentives.

The most recent view of intrinsic motivation considers motivation on a continuum from purely intrinsic to purely extrinsic motivation (with amotivation, no motivation at all, at one end of the continuum; see Figure 2.1). In addition, the highest level of intrinsic motivation is associated with high levels of self-determination, with amotivation and pure extrinsic motivation being associated with low levels of self-determination. Both intrinsic and extrinsic motivation are seen as multidimensional, with each construct being made up of different aspects. Specifically, intrinsic motivation is seen as being composed of participating in an activity purely for the knowledge, accomplishment, and stimulation that it provides.

Extrinsic motivation is seen as varying in the degree to which the behavior is extrinsically or intrinsically motivated. For example, people can participate in sport for purely extrinsic reasons (e.g., the only reason they play is to make money), for both intrinsic and extrinsic reasons (e.g., an athlete stays in shape in part to impress the opposite sex) or for purely intrinsic reasons (e.g., a runner trains diligently because she simply loves to run).

Intrinsic motivation and external rewards

Over the past 30 years, an interesting dilemma has appeared regarding the relationship between extrinsic rewards and intrinsic motivation. Specifically, it was originally thought that intrinsic and extrinsic motivation were additive. In essence, if athletes were intrinsically motivated to figure skate and they were given external rewards to figure skate (e.g., a big contract), then they would be more motivated to skate. However, recent research has challenged this additive notion, as it has been found that extrinsic rewards can either increase or decrease intrinsic motivation, depending on how the reward is seen. Cognitive evaluation theory holds that every reward has two functions. One is a controlling function and the other is an informational function.

Amotivation   ←→   Extrinsic motivation   ←→   Intrinsic motivation

Low self-determination   ←→   High self-determination

Types of intrinsic motivation
Stimulation: experience pleasant sensations such as fun, and excitement
Knowledge: derives from learning and trying something new
Accomplishment: experience pleasant sensations when mastering difficult skills

Types of extrinsic motivation (ranging from mostly extrinsic to mostly intrinsic motivation)
External regulation: behavior completely controlled by external sources (e.g., perform an activity solely to get rewards)
Introjected regulation: behavior motivated by internal prods, but still regulated by extrinsic concerns (e.g., exercising to stay in shape to impress the opposite sex)
Identified regulation:behavior is highly valued by the individual, but the activity is not pleasant in itself (e.g., an athlete participates in sport because she believes her involvement contributes to her development)
Integrated regulation: activity is important because of its valued outcome, rather than interest in the activity itself (e.g., an athlete trains diligently for the valued outcome of completing a marathon)

Figure 2.1. Continuum of intrinsic and extrinsic motivation

If a reward is seen as controlling one's behavior (e.g., holding a professional contract over a player's head), then that would change the cause of the behavior from internal to external (e.g., "I am doing it for the contract") and thus intrinsic motivation would decrease. Conversely, if the reward makes an athlete feel more competent and self-determining (e.g., "I received the MVP award because I was the best all-around player on the team"), then that would increase intrinsic motivation.

Although there are two potential aspects to every reward, how the reward will affect intrinsic motivation of the recipient depends on if it is perceived to be more controlling or more informational. In general, perceived choice and positive feedback brings out the informational aspects, whereas time deadlines and surveillance make the controlling aspects salient. A case in point regarding these competing aspects is seen in the following true scenario regarding a high school wrestler. This wrestler had a great deal of talent, had won most of his matches, and received positive feedbacks from coaches and teammates. In addition, as team captain, he helped in developing rules and practice regimens. Despite all of this, the wrestler lacked positive affect, persistence, and desire, which baffled the coach. Later on, the coach found out that the boy's father put considerable pressure on him to wrestle and constantly criticized him when

he felt the boy's performance was not up to par. In essence, the wrestler saw the controlling aspect emanating from his overbearing father as more important than the positive feedback and rewards he was receiving from his wrestling performance. This perceived external cause for his behavior was central in reducing his intrinsic motivation to wrestle.

Enhancing intrinsic motivation

Depending on the circumstances, external rewards can enhance or detract from one's internal motivation. There are several key ways to enhance intrinsic motivation.

Vary content and sequence of practice drills

Practices in sport can get tedious and boring. Adding variety to drills can increase fun and keep athletes more focused and interested in learning skills.

Involve participants in decision-making

Giving more responsibility to the participants for making decisions and rules adds to their feeling of personal accomplishment and involvement. Athletes might plan a new drill for practice or, if mature enough, have input into competitive/game strategy.

Use verbal and non-verbal praise

People often forget how powerful praise can be in enhancing motivation. A simple "good job" or "way to go" can go a long way to athletes feeling better about themselves and of their contribution to the team. This praise might be especially important if an athlete is in a slump or experiencing a plateau in learning or performing.

Set realistic performance goals

Winning is really out of athletes' control, but setting realistic goals in relation to their own performance is always achievable. These goals might simply be keeping emotional control, going through one's routine, or improving upon one's last performance. Reaching goals is a sign of competence and improvement, which generally help improve intrinsic motivation.

Give rewards contingent on performance

It is important to tie rewards to the performance of specific behaviors to increase their informational value. For example, rewards based on good sporting behaviors, proper execution of plays, helping other teammates, or mastering a difficult skill all provide information about the individual's competence.

Summary and conclusions

Motivation is one of the most important aspects for obtaining peak performance. However, many coaches and athletes are not aware of the research on specific strategies and techniques to enhance motivation. The focus of this chapter was to provide a sampling of some of the more important theoretical and practical information as it relates to enhancing motivation. Specifically, four areas were highlighted, including (i) goal setting, (ii) goal orientation, (iii) feedback/reinforcement, and (iv) intrinsic motivation. Application of strategies in each of these areas can boost the effort, persistence, enjoyment, and, ultimately, performance of athletes.

CASE STUDY

Athlete
The athlete was Scott, a 32-year-old male baseball player who had been in the major leagues for 10 years.

Reason for consultancy
Scott had been a highly motivated player for most of his career and worked out regularly in the off-season to stay in shape (or get in better shape) and always looked forward to Spring Training and the start of the season. But in the recent past he was starting to lose that enthusiasm and had a harder time getting himself motivated, as other things in his life (e.g., a wife and new baby) started to take on more meaning. Although obviously his wife and baby were very important to him, he felt he had a few good years of high-quality baseball left in him and wanted to make the most of them. But he was concerned about his lack of motivation and wanted to see if he could "rekindle the fire" that he naturally had at the beginning of his career.

Professional assessment
Upon assessing him both through interview and questionnaires, the sport psychology consultant found a couple of important

things regarding his motivation. First, Scott used to be very intrinsically motivated but after being successful and making a good deal of money, he sort of lost some motivation and started to become complacent. In addition, because he achieved a lot of individual success, the goals he used to have for himself did not seem that important any more and, in fact, he stopped setting goals at all. At this stage in his life, he wanted to try and regain that motivation for the next several years so when he was done with baseball he could say without reservations that he gave it his all.

Intervention
The sport psychology consultant believed that a goal setting intervention would be appropriate to get Scott back on track and prepared for the upcoming season (and seasons to come). Goal setting principles guided the intervention, which began with Scott setting a long-term goal that would help define his short-term goals. His long-term goals were to play five more seasons, stay injury-free, have a batting average of .300, and give full effort every day of the season. Of course some of these goals were more specific and measurable than others, but they did provide an overall context for what he wanted to

CASE STUDY (Continued)

accomplish. Then using goal setting principles, Scott and the sport psychology consultant devised a series of short-term goals to help him reach his long-term goals. For example, to help Scott remain injury-free, a very detailed and specific off-season physical fitness training regimen was devised with the help of a certified physical trainer and a nutritionist. The regimen included specific exercises for strength, endurance, and flexibility as well as a healthy diet. The regimen was modified during the season, but the basic elements remained the same. To achieve a batting average of .300 (he had averaged .292 thus far in his career), Scott needed to develop a more specific pre-at-bat routine as well as a routine of what to do between pitches (because he had a tendency to relive the previous pitch and not focus on the upcoming pitch). The routine started with a cue, which was to put on his batting helmet, and very specific behaviors and thoughts were developed from this point forward each time at-bat.

To help with the intrinsic motivation and enjoyable/fun aspect of playing, the sport psychology consultant asked Scott what used to make it fun and why was it not so much fun anymore. Based on his responses, the sport psychology consultant had him focus on staying positive because he had a tendency to get down on himself when he wasn't playing well or the team was floundering. In addition, the sport psychology consultant had him highlight the fact that people were paying money just to see him play and what a great and unique opportunity to be in a position as a successful major league baseball player that millions dream of, but very few actually achieve. Finally, Scott and the sport psychology consultant tried to make sure that in addition to preparing to play, he did things he enjoyed, such as spending time with his wife and child in the off-season and changing up his routine to avoid boredom.

Outcome

In the 2-year period after setting goals with the sport psychology consultant and initiating changes to enhance intrinsic motivation, Scott thrived and achieved most of his goals. He stayed on a strict training and dietary regimen during both the season and the off-season, he batted .297 and .305, developed a consistent routine before batting, and enjoyed himself more as he gained a better perspective of balancing his professional baseball life and his family life.

References

Weinberg, R.S., Gould, D. (2007) *Foundations of Sport and Exercise Psychology*, 4th Edn. Human Kinetics, Champaign, IL.

Further reading

Burton, D., Naylor, S., Holliday, B. (2001) Goal setting in sport: investigating the goal effectiveness paradigm. In R. Singer, H. Hausenblas & C. Janelle (eds.) *Handbook of Sport Psychology,* 2nd Edn, pp. 497–528. Wiley, New York.

Harwood, C. (2005) Goals: more than just the score. In S. Murphy (ed.) *The Sport Psych Handbook*, pp. 19–36. Human Kinetics, Champaign, IL.

Locke, E., Latham, G. (2002) Building a practically useful theory of goal setting and task performance. *American Psychologist* **57**, 705–717.

Martin, G., Hrycaiko, D. (1983) *Behavior Modification and Coaching: Principles, Procedures, and Research*. Charles C. Thomas, Springfield, IL.

Ryan, R., Deci, E. (2000) Self-determination theory and the facilitation of intrinsic motivation, social development, and well-being. *American Psychologist* **55**, 68–78.

Weinberg, R., Butt, J. (2005) Goal setting in sport and exercise domains: the theory and practice of effective goal setting. In D. Hackfort, J. Duda & R. Lidor (eds.) *Handbook of Research in Applied Sport and Exercise Psychology: International Perspectives*, pp. 129–146. Fitness Information Technology, Morgantown, WVA.

Chapter 3
Attention, concentration and thought management

Aidan P. Moran

School of Psychology, University College, Dublin, National University of Ireland, Ireland

I have learned to cut out all the unnecessary thoughts ... on the track. I simply concentrate. I concentrate on the tangible – on the track, on the race, on the blocks, on the things I have to do. The crowd fades away and the other athletes disappear and now it's just me and this one lane (Michael Johnson, two-times Olympic gold medallist in 400 m, and nine-times a world athletics gold medalist).

(Miller, 1997)

Everything is about concentration and that's what I've learnt this season. We have a great team and we're always on the attack so our opponents get maybe one or two chances in the game. Sometimes it can be one chance in 90 minutes and it's difficult to be concentrated for the right moment (Petr Cech—goalkeeper of Chelsea who set a record for goalkeepers by keeping 24 "clean sheets" in the English Premier League).

(Szczepanik, 2005)

Introduction

Concentration, or the ability to focus on the task at hand while ignoring distractions, is a vital determinant of successful performance in sport. One way to illustrate this claim is to consider the importance attached to this mental skill by leading athletes such as Michael Johnson (the former

Sport Psychology. 1st edition. Edited by Britton Brewer.
Published 2009 by Blackwell Publishing.
ISBN 978-1-4051-7363-6.

Olympic champion) and Petr Cech (goalkeeper for the soccer team Chelsea) in the quotations above. Additional evidence for the importance of "focusing" in sport comes from situations in which it fails or is disrupted in some way. For example, consider how the American rifle shooter Matthew Emmons squandered an opportunity to win a gold medal in the 2008 Olympic Games 50 m three-position target event due to a lapse in concentration. Leading his nearest rival Qiu Jian (China) by 3.3 points as he took his last shot, Emmons lost his focus and inexplicably misfired, ending up with a 4.4 for his efforts— and 4th place. This example shows clearly that in elite-level sport, effective concentration can mean the difference between winning and losing an Olympic gold medal.

Unfortunately, there are many unresolved issues in research on attentional processes in athletes. For example, what exactly happens in our minds when we "concentrate" on something? Why do athletes "lose" their concentration so easily? What kinds of distractions are encountered in competitive sport? What psychological principles govern an optimal focus in sport? And perhaps most importantly of all, what practical techniques can athletes use in order to improve their focusing skills and thinking habits in competitive situations? The purpose of this chapter is to answer these and other important questions about attention, concentration, and thought management. Before doing so, however, the distinction between attention and concentration needs to be clarified.

Attention and concentration

Contemporary cognitive psychologists regard the mind as a limited-capacity information processing system. One reason for this limitation is that people's working memory or current awareness is very brief and fragile. To explain, psychologists distinguish between "long-term memory" (an unconscious system designed to store vast amounts of information for indefinite periods of time) and "working memory" (a conscious system that people use whenever they store and manipulate currently relevant information such as the name of someone you have been introduced to at a party or a telephone number given to you verbally) for a short period of time. Unless information that enters working memory is deliberately rehearsed, it will be lost forever within 15–30 s. Given this limitation, a crucial challenge that the mind faces is how to cope with the abundance of information available to it not only from the external world, but also from the internal world of people's memories and imaginations. This task is made easier by a cognitive process called "attention," a mental process that prevents information overload by facilitating the selection of some stimulation for further processing while inhibiting that of other stimulation. Research on attention is one of the most important fields in cognitive psychology and cognitive neuroscience, because it addresses the issue of how voluntary control and subjective experience arise from, and interact with, everyday behavior. But what exactly does the term "attention" mean?

In psychology, attention is a paradoxical concept because it is familiar yet mysterious. How can this be? Well, on the one hand, it is a *familiar* term because it is ubiquitous in people's everyday language. To illustrate, a hockey coach may ask her athletes to "pay attention" to something important that she is about to say before a game. Based on an intuitive understanding of this process of focusing in daily life, William James (1890) observed famously that

> *Everyone knows what attention is.* It is the taking possession by the mind, in clear and vivid form, of one of what may seem several simultaneously possible objects or trains of thought. Focalization, concentration, of consciousness are of its essence. *It implies withdrawal from some things in order to deal effectively with others* (italics added).

On the other hand, attention is also a rather mysterious concept because it is multidimensional, with at least three different component processes. To begin with, at an experiential level, the attentional process of "concentration" refers to people's deliberate investment of conscious mental effort in processing information that is important to them at a given moment. For example, a swimmer displays "concentration" when she makes a big effort to listen carefully to every word of her coach's instructions before a big race. The second dimension of attention involves selective perception or the ability to "zoom in" on task-relevant information while ignoring potential distractions. For example, penalty takers in soccer have to learn to focus only on the ball as they place it on the penalty spot while ignoring the distracting movements of the goalkeeper or other players. The third attentional process is "divided attention" and refers to the fact that with sufficient practice, athletes can learn to perform two or more concurrent actions equally well. For example, a basketballer can dribble with the ball and scan the court for possible passing opportunities while running at speed. In summary, attention involves at least three different dimensions—the deliberate investment of mental effort, selective perception, and a form of mental time-sharing on which people can perform two or more skills equally well. The remainder of this chapter will be devoted mainly to the first of these dimensions of attention—namely the process of concentration.

Concentration as a mental spotlight: The practical value of a good metaphor

A famous psychologist named Kurt Lewin once remarked that there is nothing so practical as a good theory. This intriguing idea is relevant when considering the importance of the spotlight meta-phor of concentration in sport psychology. Before this metaphor is introduced, however, some back-ground information is necessary. Briefly, scientists have always tried to explain the *unknown* in terms of the *known*. For example, prior to the advent of information processing psychology, the memory system was often compared to a container. This metaphor was challenged, however, by research findings showing that the more one *knows*, the more one can remember. And since the mind expands to accommodate new information, the "container" metaphor of memory fell into disre-pute. So, what metaphors best capture the essence of concentration? A useful way to understand this important cognitive process is to imagine it as a *mental spotlight* that one shines at things that attract one's interest. This spotlight is like the head-mounted torches that miners or divers wear in dark environments. Wherever they direct their gaze, their target is illuminated and reaches conscious awareness. When people's absorption in a target reaches a point where there is no difference between what people are thinking about and what they are doing, then they are said to be truly "focused." Interestingly, this type of peak experience can occur only if the performer concentrates on actions that are specific, relevant to the task at hand and, above all, under his or her own control. This point will be reiterated later in the chapter.

The spotlight metaphor of attention has sev-eral advantages for athletes and coaches. Firstly, it highlights the fact that, despite what people say in everyday situations, concentration is never really "lost" but merely directed at the "wrong" target—something that is irrelevant to the task at hand (e.g., the behavior of the crowd) or that is distracting for athletes because it makes them think too far ahead (e.g., when wondering about the possible result of a game long before it is over). Secondly, the spotlight metaphor is helpful in persuading sport perform-ers that no matter what happens, they always have considerable control over what they pay attention to in any situation. Specifically, they can change the direction or width of their mental beam. To explain, at any given moment, they can direct their spotlight outward at people or objects in their environment, thereby showing an *external* focus of attention. This

happens, for example, when a sprinter listens care-fully for the sound of the gun at the start of a race. Alternatively, athletes can choose an *internal* focus of attention by deliberately concentrating on their own thoughts, feelings, or bodily processes. For example, many elite marathon runners make a deliberate effort to listen to their breathing or to focus on the rhythm of their stride in an effort to counter-act feelings of pain or fatigue that affect athletes in such endurance events. Interestingly, emerging evi-dence in sport psychology suggests that the accu-racy of a sport skill depends significantly on what the performer focuses on while executing it. More precisely, it seems that an *external* focus of attention (i.e., one in which the performers concentrate on the effects of their movements on the environment) is usually superior to an *internal* focus of atten-tion (where performers focus on their own body or on the mechanics of the action) when learning or performing sport skills. Apparently, this princi-ple holds true across a variety of skills and levels of sporting expertise. Another feature of an athlete's mental spotlight is that it has an adjustable beam. Expanding this beam allows athletes to absorb lots of information rapidly, whereas narrowing it ena-bles them to concentrate on just one thought. This "one thought" principle is one of the factors gov-erning an effective focus in sport and is addressed later in the chapter.

To summarize, the spotlight metaphor of attention suggests that athletes' minds are always focused on a target, whether external or internal. More precisely, depending on the direction and width of a person's mental spotlight, his or her concentration at any given moment falls into any one of four categories—broad external, broad internal, narrow external, or narrow internal. Of course, whether or not an ath-lete's focus is *appropriate* for the skill that he or she is performing is a very different question. For example, research shows that thinking technically about one's skills while executing them is unhelpful because it can induce a form of "paralysis by analysis" in which normally automatic processes become labored and complex. Likewise, shining one's spotlight on *oneself* is not a good idea as it makes one self-conscious and can lead to performance difficulties. And this finding raises an important question: Why do athletes seem to lose their concentration so easily?

Why do athletes "lose" their concentration?

It has long been known that skilled athletes allow their minds to wander and find it difficult to stay in the present moment in competitive situations. What psychological factors underlie this cognitive weakness? Research shows that people's concentration system is inherently fragile as a result of a combination of evolutionary and psychological factors. From an evolutionary perspective, our ancestors' survival depended on their ability to concentrate for a period of time that was sufficiently long to enable them to learn new skills. However, the capacity to monitor danger in the environment while concentrating on skill learning was also adaptive. How else could people survive the threat of being attacked by predators? Clearly, a certain degree of distractibility was probably "hardwired" into our ancestors' brains to prevent them from being completely absorbed in every task that they performed. A second reason for people's limited concentration span stems from the design of working memory—the mental blackboard (mentioned earlier) that provides a temporary and accessible workspace for us in our daily lives. This memory system regulates conscious attention by holding a small amount of information in mind for a matter of seconds. To illustrate the fragility of this system, have you ever found yourself walking into a room in your house to look for something but forgetting what it was as soon as you walked through the door? If people forget their intentions so readily, what hope do they have of remaining focused for an entire sporting event in the face of pressure and distractions? A practical strategy for dealing with this problem will be considered later in this chapter when outlining the use of "trigger words" as concentration techniques. In summary, athletes allow their minds to drift partly because of hardwired design features of the mind and partly because they allow distractions to become the target of their mental spotlight. So, what kinds of distractions are encountered in competitive sport?

Understanding distractions in sport

Although distractions take various forms, they can be divided into two main categories depending on their origin—"external" and "internal." By way of clarification, external distractions are objective environmental events and situations that divert athletes' attention away from its intended target. In contrast, internal distractions are largely subjective factors and include athletes' own thoughts, feelings, and/or bodily sensations that may hamper their efforts to concentrate on the job at hand.

Typical external distractions include factors such as crowd noise or spectator movements, sudden changes in background noise levels, gamesmanship by opponents, and unpredictable playing surfaces or weather conditions. For example, some soccer teams playing against the Turkish football club, Galatasaray, in the Ali Sami Yen stadium in Istanbul, have complained of being greeted by hostile supporters letting off fireworks and waving threatening banners bearing hostile messages such as "Welcome to hell!" Not surprisingly, these intimidating gestures make it difficult for opposing teams to focus properly before matches. The behavior of spectators can also be distracting. To illustrate, consider a strange event that occurred during the marathon race in the 2004 Olympic Games in Athens. As the Brazilian athlete Vanderlei De Lima led the field about 36 km into the race, a spectator (an eccentric priest who was subsequently defrocked) jumped out at him from the footpath and wrestled him to the ground, thereby impeding his progress. Naturally, De Lima was shocked and distracted by this assault, but regained his composure quickly to return to the race. Nevertheless, he ended up in third place behind the eventual winner, Stefano Baldini of Italy. Bad weather can also be distracting. For example, in the Wimbledon championship of 2007, the Australian tennis player Lleyton Hewitt complained about the distractions posed by rain delays before his match against Guillermo Canas (Argentina). They warmed up an estimated 10–15 times and actually started their match at least six times before it was eventually played—a remarkably distracting set of circumstances. Another classic external distraction is caused by gamesmanship from opponents. For example, taunting opponents is rampant in team games. For example, in the 2006 World Cup soccer final, with the teams at 0–0, the French player Zinedine Zidane was sent off for retaliating physically to a jibe uttered by his Italian opponent Marco Materazzi. Tellingly, Italy went on to win the game. Another example of gamesmanship in timed physical contact sports occurs when players try to "run down the clock" and break the momentum of a game by faking or exaggerating injuries. Another distracting ploy occurs widely in soccer when the opposing team's forwards often stand in front of the goalkeeper in an effort to prevent him/her from tracking the flight of the incoming ball. Regrettably, gamesmanship is also apparent in non-contact sports. To illustrate, some tennis players have been accused of "legalized cheating" because of their habit of grunting and screaming during rallies—a tactic that prevented opponents from hearing the ball coming off the strings of their rackets. Interestingly, Maria Sharapova's screams on court have been estimated to be louder than the noise created by a pneumatic drill!

As mentioned earlier, internal distractions include any thoughts, emotions (e.g., anger), and/or bodily sensations (e.g., pain, fatigue) that prevent people from concentrating fully on the job at hand. One of the most common of these distractions comes either from thinking about past mistakes or from thinking too far ahead—wondering about what will happen in the future rather than focusing on what one has to do right now. Other such distractions include thinking about the result of a match long before it is over, worrying about what other people (e.g., a coach) might say or do during a sports contest, and feeling tired or upset emotionally.

Sometimes, these distractions combine in subtle ways to disrupt athletes' concentration. To illustrate, consider how the Republic of Ireland soccer team narrowly failed to qualify automatically for the Euro 2000 international football tournament. They led Macedonia 1–0 in Skopje, Macedonia, as the match was in the third minute of injury time. At that point, an Irish player asked the referee how long was left and was told that there were only about 10 s to go. Suddenly, a corner kick was awarded to Macedonia. As the ball came into the Irish penalty area, none of the Irish players noticed a Macedonian defender running from midfield. He headed the ball into the Irish net for an equalizing goal. Obviously, asking the referee how long was left was a lapse in concentration and distracted the Irish player who should have been marking the Macedonian "runner" from midfield. Interestingly, fatigue probably compounded this error as more goals tend to be scored in the *final* 10–15 min of a game than at any other time in a soccer match.

Athletes' views of concentration and distractions

Having explained the theoretical distinction between external and internal distractions in sport, it may be helpful to explore athletes' views about concentration and distractions (see Table 3.1).

Table 3.1 Exploring distractions in sport (based on Moran, 2004).

The main purpose of this exercise is to find out what the term "concentration" means to athletes. In addition, it will help to identify various distractions that athletes experience in their sport and will explore how these distractions affect their performance.

Here are some questions to ask to elite athletes:
1. What does the term "concentration" mean to you?
2. On a scale of 0 (meaning "not at all important") to 5 (meaning "extremely important"), how important do you think that the skill of concentration is for successful performance in your sport?
3. If you think that concentration is important, do you allocate any time each week in training to developing this skill? If not, why?
4. What distractions tend to upset your concentration *before* a performance? Describe the situation and the distractions that result from it.
5. What distractions bother you *during* the event itself? Again, describe the situation and the distraction that results from it.
6. Thinking of a recent competition, give me a specific example of how a distraction changed your focus and/or affected your performance. Tell me what the distraction was, how it occurred, and how you reacted to it.
7. Do you use any specific techniques for dealing with distractions? Please explain and give an example.

Learning points
This exercise will help you to understand what "concentration" means to athletes and to explore the practical strategies that athletes use to deal with the distractions that they experience. It will also indicate whether or not athletes devote any time per week to actually improving their focusing skills.

In reply to the questions contained in Table 3.1, athletes usually indicate that concentration is very important for success in sport, but that they rarely devote any training time to improving this skill in any given week.

In addition to this practical neglect of concentration skills, it is disappointing to discover that little research has been conducted on athletes' *experience* of distractions. This neglect of the phenomenology of distractibility is largely due to two factors—one theoretical and the other methodological. The theoretical factor is that for many years, cognitive researchers falsely assumed that information flows into the mind in only one direction—inward from the outside world. In accepting this assumption, researchers have ignored the possibility that information could travel in the opposite directions, that is, from long-term memory into working memory. A second reason for the neglect of internal distractions in psychology has its roots in a methodological bias. To explain, researchers focused on external distractions simply because they were easier to measure than were self-generated distractions. As a result of this bias, few studies have been conducted on the theoretical mechanisms by which internal distractions disrupt concentration processes in athletes.

Principles of effective concentration

Based on the relevant research literature, at least five theoretical principles of effective concentration in sport may be identified. Three of them describe the establishment of an optimal focus, whereas the other two indicate how it may be disrupted (Figure 3.1).

Athletes have to decide to concentrate: It does not happen by chance

The first principle of effective concentration is the idea that one has to make a *deliberate* decision to invest mental effort in some aspect of one's athletic performance. In short, athletes have to *prepare* to concentrate rather than hope that it will happen by chance. One way in which sport performers can implement this principle is to establish an imaginary "switch on" zone before their performance. For example, as soon as some athletes enter the locker room before a game, they mentally engage their concentration system as if flicking on a switch. This idea of learning to turn one's concentration on and off takes a lot of practice, however.

Athletes can concentrate on only one thought at a time

A second principle of effective concentration is the "one thought" notion—the idea that athletes (just like everyone else) can focus consciously on only *one thing* at a time. Although people can learn to do several things at the same time, the fragility of their working memory system (explained earlier) means that they can think of only one thing at any given moment. In sport, athletes often develop such a form of single-mindedness as a response to a specific turning point or influential incident in their career. For example, Bjorn Borg, the Swedish tennis genius with the ice-cool temperament who won five consecutive Wimbledon championships, revealed that he had not always been as calm as he had appeared in competitive matches:

> When I was twelve, I behaved badly on court, swearing, cheating, throwing rackets—so my club suspended me for six months. When I came back, I didn't open my mouth ... I felt that I played my best tennis being focused and concentrating.
>
> (Hodge, 2000)

Athletes' minds are focused when there is no difference between what they are doing and what they are thinking

A third principle of effective concentration is the idea that one's mind is truly focused when one is so absorbed in the task at hand that there is no difference between one's actions and thoughts. This fusion of body and mind is especially characteristic of peak performance experiences. For example, after Roger Bannister had run the first sub-4-minute mile in May 1954 in Oxford, he said: "There was no pain,

1. Athletes have to *decide* to concentrate
   — it will not happen by chance

2. Athletes can concentrate on only
   one thought at a time

3. Athletes' minds are focused
   when there is *no difference*
   between what they are doing
   and what they are thinking

4. Athletes *lose* their concentration when
   they focus on factors that are outside
   their control

5. Athletes should *focus outwards* when they get
   nervous

Figure 3.1. Concentration principles
(based on Moran, 1996, 2004)

only a great unity of movement and aim" (Bannister, 2004, p. 12). Similarly, when Britain's David Hemery won a gold medal in the 400m hurdles in the Olympic Games in Mexico city, he explained the remarkable fusion of his mind and body:

> Only a couple of times in my life have I felt in such condition that my mind and body worked as one. This was one of those times. My limbs reacted as my mind was thinking: total control, which resulted in absolute freedom. Instead of fording and working my legs, they responded with the speed and in the motions that were being asked of them.
>
> (S. Jones, 1995)

Research suggests that the best way to increase one's chances of achieving this state of mind is to concentrate on actions that are specific, relevant, and, above all, under one's own control.

Athletes lose their concentration when they focus on factors that are outside their control

The fourth principle suggests that athletes are most likely to lose their focus whenever they concentrate on factors that are outside their control, irrelevant to the job at hand, or that have not yet happened. For example, Pete Sampras, the former US tennis champion who holds the record for the greatest number of Grand Slam titles victories achieved to date (15), lost his momentum in the Australian Open final in 1994 when serving for the match at 5–2 in the third set against Todd Martin. He double-faulted and lost the next two games mainly because he began to think too far ahead:

> I was thinking about winning the Australian Open and what a great achievement, looking ahead and just kind of taking it for granted instead of taking it point by point.
>
> (Roberts, 1994)

Despite losing his momentum, Sampras regained his concentration and went on to win the set and the match.

Athletes should focus outward when they get nervous

The final building block of effective concentration is the proposition that when athletes get nervous, they should focus *outward* on actions and not inward on doubts. This switch to an external focus is necessary because anxiety tends to make people self-critical and "hypervigilant" (i.e., excessively sensitive to any sign of what they dread). Interestingly, recent research suggests that athletes' focus of attention affects the quality and accuracy of their skills. More precisely, there is growing evidence that athletes who focus *outward*, concentrating on the effects of their actions, tend to perform better than counterparts who display an internal focus of attention (i.e., who concentrate on themselves or on the mechanics of their skills). This advice makes sense because when athletes concentrate on the mechanics of their skills, they are likely to experience a sudden deterioration in performance known as "paralysis by analysis".

Having identified some key principles of effective concentration, it is now important to consider how these ideas can be implemented by athletes in practical terms.

Practical concentration techniques and tips on thought management

Lots of techniques are available to help athletes to focus properly. The ones that are described in the following are effective mainly because they are based on the principle that optimal performance emerges when there is no gap between what athletes are doing and what they are thinking.

(i) Setting performance goal: Focusing on actions not results

Sport psychologists distinguish between outcome goals (e.g., the results of a game) and performance goals (i.e., actions that serve as stepping stones to results). Armed with this distinction, many athletes set performance goals in an effort to improve their concentration. For example, a swimmer may focus completely on making a good start before a race. Similarly, a tennis player may set himself the goal of getting at least 75% accuracy on his first serve in a match. The rationale underlying this strategy is that by focusing on actions that are under one's own control, one is less likely to be distracted than if one allows oneself to think too far ahead.

(ii) Using routines

A second concentration technique involves the use of "pre-performance routines" or consistent sequences of thoughts and actions that athletes display before executing key skills. Psychologically, routines are valuable because they take athletes seamlessly from thinking about something to actually doing it. They improve concentration because they help sports performers to focus on the job that they have to do, one step at a time. For example, top tennis players tend to bounce the ball a certain number of times before serving. Also, by concentrating on each step of one's routine, athletes ensure that they stay in the present moment.

Routines are extensively used by top athletes. For example, the British 2004 Olympic champion Kelly Holmes revealed the routine that led her to double-gold medal success at the Games in Athens:

> After the first heat of the 800m, the races were always around the same time so I stuck to the same routine. I left for the track at the same time, I kept wearing my Team GB dog-tag around my neck, and it became my lucky charm, kissing it. When I went to the warm-up track, I would listen to Alicia Keys singing "If I ain't got you" and applied the words to the gold medal I wanted. I sang it as I warmed up and it brought tears to my eyes because I was dreaming of a gold medal. When I eventually got it, I kept the same routine for the 1500m. I cried before I left to run the 800m final because it was either going to be my dream or it would go all wrong and I cried again before the 1500m—I have been an emotional wreck.
>
> (Mackay, 2004)

(iii) Using "trigger words"

A third focusing technique involves the use of trigger words or short, vivid, and positively phrased verbal reminders designed to help athletes to focus on a specific target or to perform a relevant action. To illustrate, during the 2002 Wimbledon ladies' singles tennis final between the Williams sisters, Serena Williams (who defeated Venus Williams 7–6, 6–3) read prepared notes to herself during the "change-over" time between games. Afterwards, she explained that she had been written certain trigger words as instructional cues to remind her to "hit in front of you" or "stay low." She also used the same technique in her fourth round defeat of Daniela Hantuchova at the 2007 Wimbledon championship, this time reminding herself to "add spin" and "move up."

(iv) Imaging what one wants to do next

A fourth concentration strategy in sport involves the use of mental imagery or "seeing" and "feeling" oneself performing a given skill in one's mind's eye before actually doing it. Imagery helps athletes to prepare for various imaginary scenarios, thereby ensuring that they will not be distracted by any unexpected events. It is also valuable in helping athletes to distinguish between "on" and "off" zones in competitive sport situations.

Imagery is widely used in sport as a concentration technique. For example, before Roger Bannister broke the 4-minute mile in 1954, he used visualization as a preparation technique: "Each night in the week before the race there came a moment when I saw myself at the starting line … I ran the race over in my mind" (Bannister, 2004, p. 12). Similarly, US athlete Mike Powell visualized all the details of his long-jump performance before setting a new record for this event at the World Track and Field Championships in Tokyo in 1991:

> Before the last jump, I knew what was going to happen … I saw it all in my mind, but this time it was like precognition: the good speed on the runway, the good timing and good takeoff on the board, that super extra burst of strength. It really was eerie.
>
> (Clarkson, 1999)

(v) Physically relaxing and centering one's body

Physical relaxation techniques can help athletes to concentrate effectively. In particular, lowering one's shoulders, doing gentle neck-rolling exercises, flapping out the tension from one's arms and legs, and taking slow deep breaths can lower one's center of gravity (a process called "centering") and reduce the likelihood of error. Interestingly, one of the biggest mistakes made by novice golfers or tennis players is to hold in their breath while they prepare for a shot. When this happens, their muscles tense up and their swing becomes jerky and inconsistent. By contrast, exhaling while relaxing the muscles is widely used as a focusing technique in sport by stars such as Darrell Pace, the former US two-times Olympic champion archer who revealed that he used to use controlled breathing as a preparation strategy before competitions. Specifically, he synchronized the pattern of his inhalations and exhalations with covert repetition of the word "relax" in an effort to improve his concentration skills.

(vi) Simulation training: Trying a dress rehearsal

Simulation training is based on the assumption that athletes will learn to concentrate more effectively in real-life pressure situations if they can re-create these situations in practice and train under them. For example, Darrell Pace used to practice shooting arrows near railroad racks and highways in an effort to simulate the distracting conditions that he experienced in competitive situations. Similarly, Dan O'Brien, the US champion who won a gold medal and set a new record for the decathlon at the 1996 Games in Atlanta, used simulation techniques over a 4-year period in order to overcome a debilitating bout of performance anxiety. Briefly, following his unexpected failure to qualify for the 1992 Olympic Games due to a sudden attack of nervousness during the US trials earlier that year, O'Brien was advised by a sport psychologist to build simulation strategies into his training program for the various decathlon events. For example, for the pole-vault, he trained in the Olympic Stadium so that he could become accustomed to the sights and sounds he would experience in that venue. In addition, O'Brien learned to contend with distractions that had been introduced deliberately by his sport psychologist during these practice sessions. Simulation training is also used in other sports such as boxing and soccer. To illustrate, the renowned trainer Brendan Ingle used to call his fighters derogatory names (e.g., "Paki" if they were Asian or "Paddy" if they were Irish) while sparring with them in order to prepare them for the verbal taunting that they would receive against certain competitive opponents in the ring.

Simulation techniques are also widely used by soccer coaches. To illustrate, Jose Mourinho, the manager who guided FC Porto to European Champions' league victory in 2004 and who subsequently won several Premier league titles with Chelsea in England, devised training drills for his players that simulated the decision-making situations (e.g., passing under pressure from opponents) that they would face in competitive matches. More generally, a list of possible simulation techniques for counteracting distractions in soccer is provided in Table 3.2.

Unfortunately, as with any simulation, there are always "fidelity" issues or doubts about the extent to which dress rehearsals can ever fully replicate the actual experience of competitive action. Having examined some popular concentration strategies used by athletes, the next topic to address is thought management in sport.

Some tips on thought management in sport

A key theme of this chapter is the idea that effective concentration requires thinking only about what one can control. But what exactly *can* athletes control in competitive sport?

Three factors stand out immediately—how they prepare for a competition, how they perform in it, and above all, how they react to mistakes and adversity during the event itself. It is usually in relation to this last point that athletes' thinking goes awry. For example, if athletes expect to play flawlessly all the time, their perfectionistic standards will prevent them from fulfiling their potential. Why? To answer briefly, it is because competitive sport always represents a compromise between what is *desirable* (e.g., playing without errors) and what is *possible* in the circumstances (e.g., minimizing the impact of an error by letting go of it so that it does not affect the next decision one makes). In this regard, Table 3.3 presents some practical tips on managing one's thoughts in the face of setbacks.

Table 3.2 Simulation techniques used in soccer coaching.

Distraction	Possible simulation technique
Crowd noise	Playing specially recorded CDs of crowd noise during training sessions in order to familiarize players with expected distractions during matches in "away" venues
Gamesmanship	Arranging for teammates to simulate opponents' possible gamesmanship (e.g., verbal insults) during training sessions or practice matches
Fatigue	Alternating normal training sessions with short bouts of high-intensity exercise in order to induce the type of fatigue that may be expected in competitive matches
Heat/humidity	Arranging for players to train and play while wearing layers of extra clothing in order to simulate hot weather conditions
Unfavorable refereeing decisions	Designing "modified" game situations containing deliberately unfair umpiring decisions
One player missing	Creating pressure situations in training (e.g., practicing the retention of possession of the ball with only 10 players) in order to simulate a situation in which one player has been sent off

Table 3.3 Reframing sport mistakes: Practical tips on thought management.

• Athletes need to be aware that although striving for perfection is a good thing, judging themselves harshly because they did not produce a perfect performance is damaging psychologically because it can erode one's confidence and self-esteem.
• Athletes must learn to avoid the habit of taking failure personally. All athletes make mistakes—but not all athletes blame themselves as a result.
• Athletes need to get their disappointments in perspective: In a year's time, they probably will not even *remember* why they were so upset about a silly mistake.
• Athletes have to avoid thinking about what might have been. Wishful (or "counterfactual") thinking cannot change anything and is a waste of time.
• Top athletes rarely focus on the mistakes they have made. Instead, they concentrate on what they plan to do differently the next time.
• Athletes can learn a great deal from the way in which successful people handle setbacks. In general, successful people try hard not to make the same mistake twice.
• Athletes should ask themselves what aspects of the setback they can change in the future: Successful people see setbacks as caused by things that they can change.
• Athletes should develop the habit of identifying at least one good thing (e.g., a lesson learned such as a change in perspective) that came out of the mistake or setback that they experienced.

The purpose of the cognitive mistake management techniques discussed earlier is to help prevent athletes from engaging in what psychologists call "snowball thinking," whereby an error in performance triggers a chain of irrelevant negative thoughts (e.g., "Typical! Another stupid mistake— I'm playing very poorly") that not only distract the athlete involved but also encourage him or her to make pessimistic predictions about the chances of winning the game or event (e.g., "I'm making so many mistakes today that I'm bound to lose"). This type of loose, unfocused thinking is the direct opposite of the "one thought" concentration principle outlined earlier.

To conclude this chapter, the relationship between concentration and thought management can be summarized as follows. If athletes can be trained to narrow their mental spotlight so that they think only about jobs that are under specific, relevant, and under their control, they have created the right frame of mind to perform to the best of their ability. Of course, this is a difficult challenge for any performer, but with appropriate training and practice, athletes can learn to improve their concentration and thinking skills. After all, as modern cognitive psychology has shown, there is no such thing as a truly difficult task—only an *unpractised* one.

CASE STUDY

Athlete

Paul is a 15-year-old tennis player who has great natural ability but whose competitive performance is inconsistent, especially during matches in which he has built up a big lead and seems close to victory. In discussion with his coach, he admits that his difficulties stem from a tendency to "lose focus" when trying to close out matches in competitive situations. For example, in a recent tournament, he was leading against his opponent when serving in the final set tiebreak, but made the mistake of thinking too far ahead—wondering who he'd be playing in the next round. This lapse in concentration led to several double faults, produced lots of negative thinking, and eventually cost him the match. Paul's coach gives another example of this problem by reporting that Paul lost four games in a row recently when leading 5–2 in the third set. In two of these games, he served several double faults, which made him very angry with himself. Fortunately, on this occasion, Paul eventually won the tiebreak mainly because his opponent made even more errors than he did. But having experienced this "wandering mind" problem a number of times in the past few months, Paul and his coach wondered what can be done about it. The urgency of the consultation comes from the fact that Paul is about to take part in a series of trial matches for a place on the national junior elite tennis squad and is very anxious to get some help. So, with 3 weeks to go, Paul and his coach have approached a sport psychologist for practical advice on preparing for matches and for concentrating effectively on court.

Reason for consultancy

Paul is not performing consistently to his full potential, is finding it hard to close out matches, and seems to have developed the habit of allowing his mind to wander when he should be focusing on the point at hand.

Intervention

Following discussions with Paul and his coach, analysis of Paul's match statistics over the previous 6 months, and observation of videotapes of several of his recent competitive performances, the sport psychologist devised a program of psychological strategies designed to improve Paul's concentration and thought management skills before and during his matches. This intervention program lasted several weeks. First, the sport psychologist trained Paul to prepare mentally for competitive matches by showing him how to "switch on" his concentration before the game itself. When sitting by himself in the locker room for a few moments prior to the warm-up, Paul was shown how to close his eyes and "see" and "feel" himself serving and returning the ball smoothly and covering the court energetically. Then, having left the locker room, Paul was shown how to switch on his mental spotlight as soon as he stepped onto the court. In particular, he was encouraged to imagine the space behind the baseline as his "switch on" zone. By stepping back toward the fence, he could switch off his concentration and by approaching the baseline he could switch it on again. Next, the psychologist trained Paul and his coach to use a number of practical concentration techniques during matches. These involved setting "performance goals" for every rally (e.g., focusing on getting his first serve wide or making a deep return), using "pre-serve routines" (e.g., steadying himself at the service line, bouncing the ball three times, visualizing his target, and then tossing the ball and serving) and reminding himself to stay focused by using silent "trigger words" inside his head (e.g., "bounce … hit" or "cross court") from time to time. At changeovers between games, Paul was also shown how to imagine himself beginning the next point strongly and confidently. He was also trained to lower his shoulders and to breathe deeply during breaks in play and to "flap" out the tension in his arms whenever he felt himself getting

CASE STUDY (Continued)

nervous. Finally, the sport psychologist and coach trained Paul to "close out" simulated game situations in which he was leading 5–3 and serving for the match. These simulated competitive situations were helpful in teaching Paul to enjoy the challenge of finishing a match with the same confidence and vigor as he had started it.

Outcome

Although Paul found it difficult to implement some aspects of the intervention program initially (e.g., he had some trouble finding a quiet time before matches as the locker room was invariably quite full and noisy), his confidence grew as he began to achieve more consistency in his performance on court. In particular,

he found that setting performance goals and using pre-serve routines helped him to concentrate effectively regardless of how well his opponent played. This newfound consistency was especially evident when he won a number of tournament matches in straight sets against lower-ranked opponents he had previously struggled to beat in three sets. Paul's coach was very pleased with the fact that Paul is now playing consistently better in tournaments than he had done before the intervention began. Slowly but surely, Paul is making progress in displaying the talent that he possesses. Perhaps most importantly of all, both Paul and his coach now know what to do when Paul experiences occasional mental lapses on court. They realize that although tennis is played with the body, it is won mainly by the mind.

References

Bannister, R. (2004) Fear of failure haunted me right to the last second. *The Guardian* (Sport) 1 May, 12–13.

Clarkson, M. (1999) *Competitive Fire*. Human Kinetics, Champaign.

Hodge, K. (2000) *Sports Thoughts*. Reed, Auckland.

James, W. (1890) *Principles of Psychology*. Holt, Rinehart and Winston, New York.

Jones, S. (1995) Inside the mind of perfection. *The Independent* (Sport) 11 December, 10.

Mackay, D. (2004) Holmes finds self-belief and double delight. *The Guardian* 30 August, 6–7.

McCarra, K. (2004) How Chelsea's "big brains" made his mark. *The Guardian* (Sport) 11 December, 1–2.

Miller, B. (1997) *Gold Minds: The Psychology of Winning in Sport*. The Crowood Press, Marlborough, Wiltshire.

Roberts, J. (1994) Sampras leaves Melbourne with his sights set firmly on Paris. *The Irish Times* 31 January, 5.

Szczepanik, N. (2005) Focused Cech puts records low on his list of priorities. *The Times* 30 April, 100.

Vealey, R.S., Walter, S.M. (1994) On target with mental skills: an interview with Darrell Pace. *The Sport Psychologist* **8**, 428–441.

Watterson, J. (1999) Paddy power *The Irish Times* (Sport) 9 January, 8.

Further reading

Kremer, J., Moran, A. (2008) *Pure Sport: Practical Sport Psychology*. Routledge/Taylor and Francis, London.

Moran, A.P. (1996) *The Psychology of Concentration in Sport Performers: A Cognitive Analysis*. Psychology Press, Hove, East Sussex.

Moran, A.P. (2004) *Sport and Exercise Psychology: A Critical Introduction*. Routledge/Psychology Press, London.

Chapter 4
Management of competitive stress in elite sport

Sheldon Hanton[1], Owen Thomas[1] and Stephen D. Mellalieu[2]

[1]Cardiff School of Sport, University of Wales Institute, Cardiff, United Kingdom
[2]Department of Sports Science, Swansea University, Swansea, United Kingdom

Introduction

One of the most studied and frequently cited areas within the field of applied sport psychology is that of competition stress and anxiety. This prominence is undoubtedly linked to the stressful nature of elite sport, and the demands associated with the competitive environments that surround the modern day performer. As a direct consequence, a core component within many athletes' competitive preparation programs includes some form of stress management focused on the achievement of an optimal pre-performance mental state.

This chapter, which contains six sections, attempts to explore these programs and provides an insight into treatment frameworks that underpin practical work with elite athletes. The opening section clarifies and places into context the key terms used within this area and outlines their importance for applied work. The second section provides an overview of the stressors (i.e., demands) that performers commonly encounter, and illustrates the types of anxiety responses athletes may experience following exposure to these demands. The third section summarizes contemporary thinking on how sport psychologists believe anxiety can affect sport performance, and also illustrates how practitioners may attempt to evaluate the athlete before

Sport Psychology. 1st edition. Edited by Britton Brewer.
Published 2009 by Blackwell Publishing.
ISBN 978-1-4051-7363-6.

recommending an intervention strategy. The fourth section provides an overview of stress management interventions in elite sport that have been designed to *reduce* the intensity of anxiety symptoms that performers commonly encounter in stressful situations. Section five then details an approach to combating stress that focuses on programs that are designed to *restructure* the performers' interpretations of anxiety symptoms from negative to positive. The concluding section highlights these treatment approaches with two case study scenarios.

Clarification and contextualization of key terms

The use of stress management within the area of competition stress and anxiety has often been hindered by lack of consistency and, at times, understanding of the central terms adopted within the literature. It is not intended to provide an in-depth debate on these issues as has occurred in some recent sport psychology texts; instead, certain terms are defined and contextualized to encourage a clearer understanding of how to manage athletes' responses in pressure situations: the primary aim of this chapter.

Contemporary thinking views stress as a dynamic relationship between athletes and their practice and competition environment. Specifically, performers appraise the demands of the situation and then attempt to cope with these demands. Inherent within this approach is the perspective that performers will encounter many different demands that tax their resources and it is the athletes' perceived ability to cope with these that form the process of *stress*. If athletes feel that they cannot cope with the demands then they are then likely to experience different levels of competition *anxiety*.

The role of appraisal within the process of stress is central to the context of determining the most appropriate stress management intervention. Specifically, the *reduction* approach to stress management suggests that performers react to the demands with negative performance consequences. This point is emphasized by sprinter Kim Collins of St Kitts when talking about his background and approach to the blue ribbon 100-m event:

> There are problems with coming from a small country ... we've never had a sprinter at this level before so I'm doing something that has never been done before ... I went to an all boy's school where if you showed fear you were in trouble, track and field is no different. If you come to the line showing fear and nerves everyone will pick on you, your self-esteem and confidence are gone. I just have to be confident and relax–relaxation is very important to me.

The content of this quote helps illustrate one of the treatment frameworks and supports one school of thought in relation to the negative influence that anxiety responses can have on sport performance. Specifically, when Collins talks about the importance of attaining a relaxed state to help him cope with pressure, his thinking is aligned with the *reduce* treatment framework (i.e., striving to lower the intensity levels of anxiety symptoms an athlete experiences). However, an alternative understanding of the stress process suggests that certain athletes possess the ability to respond to the demands of competitive performance and their anxiety symptoms in a positive way. The following quote from one of the most successful swimmers in Olympic history, Australia's Ian Thorpe, helps in this respect:

> For me Sydney was a dream, as a kid that's all I ever wanted to do was swim an Olympic games.... And my ultimate dream was to win

an Olympic gold medal and I was able to achieve that in Sydney. I guess there was always a lot of attention on me, a lot of expectation on me to perform well and if you turn those into a positive thing it becomes support, whereas if you turn it into a negative thing it then becomes pressure.

Thorpe's sentiments help show the second treatment framework presented within this chapter that suggests experiencing anxiety symptoms does not always have a negative effect on performance. Specifically, when Thorpe talks about turning expectation and pressure into a positive way for performance, his thinking is aligned with the *restructuring* treatment approach adopted within contemporary stress management programs (i.e., striving to interpret anxiety symptoms in a positive way).

Competition stressors and athletes' responses

Several research studies in applied sport psychology have examined the different stressors, or demands, that performers may have to deal with in stressful situations. Here the literature suggests that aspects of competition (e.g., thinking about performance, the goals that may have been set, and perceived levels of physical and mental preparation), interpersonal relationships (e.g., expectations from teammates, coaches, family members), financial matters (e.g., funding issues, sponsors), traumatic experiences (e.g., the risk and consequence of injury), and the weather and environmental conditions can result in athletes having different anxiety responses.

An important distinction to make at this stage is the separation of anxiety into cognitive and somatic symptoms. So far, the term *anxiety* has been used in a global way to describe how performers respond to the demands within stressful situations. It is important to realize, however, that coaches and practitioners should distinguish between athletes' mental and perceived physical responses to the stressors they encounter. Specifically, cognitive anxiety responses are the thoughts athletes experience in stressful situations such as worries, negative expectations, and apprehensions about performance (i.e., athletes' mental response to stressors). However somatic responses are the athletes' perceptions of their physiological arousal state in stressful environments (i.e., athletes' perceived physical response to stressors). Symptoms categorized as somatic include muscular tension, butterflies in their stomach, increased heart rate, and perspiration. The following section helps to highlight why this distinction is important in the context of stress management interventions; specifically, the notion that within certain approaches these differing mental and physical symptoms require specific and individual psychological skill programs to be most effective. This feature applies for both the reduction and restructure frameworks. For example, within the reduction approach, a performer who experiences high physical anxieties would usually be provided with a somatic (i.e., physical) relaxation treatment, such as progressive muscle relaxation, in an attempt to align the treatment to the physical response. Within the restructure approach, performers interpreting their mental anxieties as negative for performance would often be provided with a cognitive (i.e., mental) treatment strategy, such as imagery or cognitive restructuring, in an attempt to match the treatment to the specific response of the athlete.

A final consideration that has a bearing for the practitioner when treating the effects of stress is the *activation* levels required to perform optimally. In this instance, *activation* refers to the appropriate mental and physical state that athletes need to be ready to perform. Perhaps the most effective way to illustrate this point is to consider the levels of activation required in two different tasks. For example, the desirable mental and physical state to demonstrate readiness to perform as an Olympic weight lifter is very different from the state of readiness needed to perform well as an Olympic target rifle shooter. For example, strength, power, and aggression are key determinants of performance within the gross muscular activity of weightlifting, whereas composure, control, and calmness are key factors within the fine muscular control event of target-shooting. It is clear that the two appropriate activation states fall at different ends of a continuum and that practitioners should consider these issues before designing interventions.

The relationship between anxiety and sport performance

Many different explanations have been forwarded in the research literature that attempt to account for the relationship between anxiety and performance. One approach is that increases in competition anxiety, and particularly cognitive symptoms, always have a detrimental effect on performance. This is the underpinning premise for the *reduction* approach to managing stress. Other researchers have suggested that the relationship with performance should be determined at a more individual level and that athletes possess optimal levels or zones of anxiety within which their performance will be maximized. These assertions led to interventions being individually tailored where, at certain times, reduction would be called for if the performer was too anxious, but on other occasions the practitioner may consider increasing anxiety levels to perform an energizing function. A third perspective is based on the principle that high levels of anxiety may be interpreted in a positive way and actually benefit sport performance. This notion links closely to the underlying message within Thorpe's quote presented earlier, and is fundamental to the *restructuring* approach.

How to assess anxiety symptoms

Prior to practitioners providing any form of intervention to athletes, an accurate assessment of the performers' anxiety symptoms should take place. To do this, sport psychologists typically adopt a combined approach to see how mentally and physically anxious performers may be and whether they interpret the anxiety symptoms experienced as positive or negative toward performance. This assessment often uses a combination of validated psychometric questionnaires alongside interviewing procedures with the athletes in question and their coaches. Sport psychologists may also ask performers to record their anxiety symptoms in some form of diary and, finally, may observe their behavior in stressful situations. Sport psychologists then collate and analyze this information and come to a conclusion about the intensity levels of mental and physical anxiety symptoms and whether these are interpreted in a positive or negative manner toward performance. This information then underpins the agreed treatment framework for the athlete.

A reduction approach to stress management intervention

As mentioned earlier, one approach to stress management adopts techniques that are designed to *reduce* competitive anxiety symptoms. In line with the distinction between the different cognitive and somatic anxiety symptoms, the treatment programs that are prescribed under the reduction approach can be broadly categorized into mental skills and physical skills. Although general in nature, it should be noted that this distinction has arisen from several groups of sport psychologists suggesting that the anxiety treatments they provide should target or *match* the dominant anxiety symptoms that the athlete experiences in a stressful encounter. To illustrate, this treatment perspective suggests that if the athlete's dominant anxiety response is somatic in nature (i.e., the intensity of the physical anxieties is higher than of the mental symptoms), then the treatment the practitioner should advise is a skill-focused mainly on reducing somatic symptoms, with less regard given to the cognitive symptoms experienced. Conversely, if the dominant anxiety response is a symptom associated with cognitive anxiety, a mental approach with less regard given to the treatment of any physical anxiety symptoms would be advocated. The skills outlined next are examples of techniques that would fit into this treatment framework, and, using the matching approach, coaches or sport psychology practitioners would select a treatment based on the performers' dominant anxiety responses.

The following sections detail the physical relaxation skills, mental relaxation skills, and thought-controlling techniques used under the umbrella of the *reduction* approach. These skills are described

as series of logical and progressive steps and are supplemented by a practical example in the form of a case study at the end of the chapter. To help athletes acquire the skills in question, a common learning framework is regularly adopted by applied sport psychologists. Briefly, the skills detailed here and in subsequent sections can be acquired through the following phases. First, the athlete learns the fundamentals of the skill in a stress-free environment working closely with the practitioner. Second, increasing independence from the practitioner, the athlete becomes more self-directed and begins to apply the skill in non-threatening situations. Third, the athlete is instructed to use, and also test the efficacy of the skill, in a non-sporting stressful environment. The final stage of learning and acquiring the skill involves the athlete applying the skills in increasingly demanding sporting situations: practice, warm-up, and fully competitive events.

Probably the most common application of a physical relaxation technique used to reduce athletes' somatic anxiety symptoms is the collection of psychological skills grouped under the rubric of *progressive muscle relaxation* techniques. Although these skills exist in several different forms, the most common enables performers to learn the skill of physical relaxation through a series of logical, progressive stages. The primary goal is for performers to reach an end point where the skill, and thus a relaxed physical state, can be attained very rapidly in practically any stressful situation. Traditionally, when learning the skill, athletes will advance through different stages where the amount of time it takes to achieve a relaxed state progressively decreases. During the preliminary stage of learning the skill, performers are required to systematically focus their attention on different gross muscle groups within the body, consciously tensing and relaxing to increase self-awareness of the difference between a tensed (anxious) state and a relaxed (less anxious) one. To supplement this process, athletes will usually be provided with some form of audio track that contains a set of instructions that methodically guides them through the muscle groups of their body. As with all the stages of the program, athletes will not progress to the next stage until they are proficient in the technique. Specifically, a constant and desirable state of physical relaxation needs to be achieved before the athlete can move on.

During the second stage of the program, the audio track is removed and the athlete is asked to simply relax the gross muscle groups used in the previous stage (rather than tense *and* relax). Once proficient, athletes can progress onto the third stage, where they focus on some form of cue that acts as an association-trigger to help invoke the relaxed state. This trigger can adopt several forms. For example, based on preference, athletes may condition the response through self-talk in the form of cue words such as "relax." Alternatively, they may use a physical action such as gripping the handle of their racquet in tennis. Finally, they may incorporate a trigger conditioned to the exhalation phase of their breathing.

The fourth stage of the process strives to make the skill portable and shift its use into more realistic settings. Athletes are taught to avoid tensing the muscles that are not involved in a particular movement and actively relax those that are involved in the activity (during the time prior to movement). Up to this point, athletes will have tended to hone their relaxation skills in completely non-threatening environments that are usually quiet, familiar, and comfortable. During the penultimate stage of learning the skill, performers are taught to integrate the technique into naturally occurring semi-stressful environments away from the sporting arena. This process requires athletes to take two to three deep breaths focusing on their conditioned trigger during the exhalation phase of breathing to gain an associated level of physical relaxation. Examples of where this technique may be practiced include queuing whilst shopping, when running late for a social event, or when stuck in traffic while driving. The final stage of the process involves application training whereby the athletes practice their technique in progressively stressful sporting environments. This final stage usually takes place gradually over a period of time to refine the skill in intense sporting situations.

In comparison to physical relaxation, mental relaxation techniques have received far less exposure as treatment approaches to reduce athletes' mental anxiety symptoms in the research literature. Practitioners have tended to focus on alternative cognitive strategies outside of those categorized as relaxation to reduce intensity levels of cognitive anxiety. However, *transcendental* mediation has been used as a mental relaxation technique with sports performers. This approach essentially adopts a cognitive-based framework with the underlying treatment target being more closely aligned with the mental anxiety symptoms experienced. Sport psychologists have, once again, tended to adopt a progressive learning approach to the skill of meditation in-line with the frameworks designed for physical relaxation. The goal of this approach focuses upon learning the skill of cognitive relaxation through a series of steps designed to transcend the mental state of the athlete from one of being mentally anxious to one of being mentally calm. Traditionally, when learning the meditative skill, performers progress through four stages to reach an end point where they can lower their levels of mental anxiety in a matter of seconds. The first stage involves athletes learning a general meditative technique that establishes a focus on breathing. Athletes are asked to introduce a "mantra" on each breath out, and once relaxed, count down from ten to one on each exhalation and then upwards from one to seven on each inhalation. The goal here is for performers to transcend down to a deeper level of cognitive relaxation and then actively shift back up to raise the level of consciousness. To supplement this process, athletes are often provided with an audio track that contains relaxing music and an instructional set outlining the process described earlier.

In the second stage, athletes are supplied with a second audio track that contains instruction but no relaxing music. The directions ask performers to focus on their mantra, and the counting procedure is subsequently reduced from five to one on exhalation, and then from one to three on inhalation to shorten the time it takes to achieve mental relaxation. Next, in the third stage the audio track is removed altogether and the athletes are instructed to discard all counting procedures. Athletes are then asked to concentrate on inhalation and repeat their mantra phrase on every exhalation. During this stage, athletes are also asked to transfer the skill into more realistic stressful settings (but away from sport) to reduce the mental anxieties experienced in these situations. The final stage of learning the meditative skill involves application training for the performer where athletes are asked to integrate the meditative skill into progressively stressful sport environments.

Other mental relaxation techniques to treat cognitive anxiety include calming mental imagery and autogenic training. Based on the proviso that an athlete has been trained in the use of imagery, calming imagery can be used to help reduce cognitive anxiety. When using this technique, the practitioners commonly ask the performers to imagine being in a relaxing environment such as on a warm beach with the sound of the waves lapping the shore, or lying in a field on a pleasant summer's day. Essentially, practitioners should advocate whatever images athletes personally believe will provide them with a sense of calmness and mental relaxation. Autogenic training is fundamentally a self-styled hypnosis strategy that performers can use to help produce the two physical sensations of "warmth" and "heaviness." The process occurs through six stages. In the first stage, performers use self-dialog (e.g., "my right arm is heavy") and focus their attention on the heavy feeling. Athletes then cancel this effect by physically moving the arm while focusing on their breathing. This process is then repeated across other body segments until the sensation of heaviness can be achieved throughout the entire body. The second stage of the process replicates the first except the goal is to achieve a "warmth" sensation in the limbs and body rather than a feeling of heaviness. The two processes of achieving these sensations are then combined so that the athlete can accomplish a warm and heavy sensation simultaneously. The third stage aims to regulate the athletes' heart rate through using a verbal suggestion such as "my heart rate is regular and calm," which is then added to the process of achieving a warm and heavy sensation. The fourth stage links these procedures to breathing rate and the fifth stage associates these processes to the regulation of the visceral organs through a focus on the solar plexus. Finally, the sixth stage asks performers to focus on the strategy of placing a cool cloth on their forehead to experience a cool sensation. Once all six stages are complete, athletes practice the entire sequence all the way

through using a verbal citation (or mantra) that combines each individual stage to lower cognitive anxiety. One limitation with autogenic training, however, is the length of time practitioners suggest it takes to acquire and become proficient in the skills to achieve strong and profound sensations. Specifically, reports have indicated that it may take up to 6 months to become adept in autogenic training even when practicing the skill on a daily basis.

Alternative techniques to reduce cognitive anxiety that fall outside of the classification of relaxation skills include the use of thought control techniques such as thought stopping or positive thought control. Traditionally, thought stopping involves having athletes keep a diary of the anxious thoughts they experience prior to or during performance that they consider negative and intrusive to their preparation and performance. Athletes are then instructed to identify a trigger word such as "stop" or "no" to act as a technique to block the negative thoughts. Self-talk and internal dialog is advised to be used as means for athletes to execute this approach. Caution is, however, advised with using this technique without considerable expertise because of the potentially deleterious effects of attempting to suppress anxious thoughts with the unintended effect being the literal opposite.

The cognitive skill of positive thought control should be seen as an extension to the thought-stopping process. Specifically, rather than ending the process with the reciting of a blocking trigger word, athletes are instructed to "replace" the negative thought with a positive one to develop a more positive psychological orientation. Traditionally, athletes use a diary method supplementary to those used to record negative thoughts, where they are encouraged to construct positive self-dialog statements to replace each negative thought experienced. Therefore, the full process of positive thought control requires athletes to first identify any negative thoughts experienced, block the thought using a thought-stopping trigger word, and then finally replace the negative thought with a positive thought to create a positive cognitive orientation.

A summary of the psychological skills presented so far aligns with the singular approach outlined in the introductory statement within this section.

Essentially, this approach advocates the use of these individual psychological skills as discrete treatment frameworks in-line with the athlete's dominant anxiety response (mental or physical). However, for certain sports, sport psychologists often recommend the use of combined mental and physical treatment packages. As such, practitioners and athletes are advised to select individualized combinations of mental and physical strategies in an attempt to treat the full range of anxiety symptoms athletes experience within stressful encounters.

It is important to note that the goal of these combined or integrated frameworks would still be focused on athletes reducing the intensity levels of anxiety symptoms. This raises an obvious issue in relation to the appropriate activation states required for certain sporting tasks. In particular, it is not always appropriate to focus *solely* on techniques designed to reduce competition anxiety symptoms. Indeed, the example given in the introduction helps illustrate this point. For the weightlifter, a reduction in both physical and mental anxieties may not be an appropriate strategy to create the best activation state for performance. An intervention approach based on this philosophy will potentially interfere with the suitable activation states required for optimal performance. In essence, therefore, the athlete may become too mentally or physically relaxed to perform. Consequently, some athletes may require, either generally or prior to certain specific tasks, an increase in anxiety levels to create the optimum activation state to enter the competitive arena. Several "energizing" techniques have been proposed to serve this function when performers require increased activation. Traditionally, these techniques are introduced after those skills designed to reduce anxiety symptoms because they are considered as more complex derivatives of the psychological skills. Essentially, practitioners can reverse the focus of several of the skills outlined in the reduction approach and use them in an energizing way rather than a relaxing way. For example, breathing exercises can be just as effective at producing an energized state as they are as a calming one. When teaching these skills, practitioners first ask the performers to use their breathing control techniques to gain a relaxed state. Following achievement of this state, athletes are

asked to consciously increase their breathing rate and imagine that with each inhalation and exhalation that they are increasing energy levels and reaching an optimum activation state. This breathing technique is usually combined with self-talk cues. For example, athletes might be advised to use a cue word such as "energy up" on inhalation. Additional techniques that practitioners can prescribe to increase activation levels involve the use of imagery-based skills. However, rather than using these in a calming function as outlined previously, the skills would be used as an energizing function. Specifically, practitioners ask athletes to image scenes that depict the creation of energy. Examples of images of this sort include images of trains moving slowly, gaining momentum and speed, images of heavy machinery where working parts move rapidly, images of natural forces such as powerful waves and winds, and images of animals sprinting and moving rapidly. Finally, rather than using self-talk skills with cue words associated with a relaxed state, this technique can also be applied in an energizing function. The content of the verbal dialog is all that needs to change for performers here, and practitioners would advocate the use of words such as "explode," "charge," and "power" to help facilitate the process of energizing the athletes' pre-performance activation level.

Unless the activation demands of the task are considered, the approach of generalizing treatments across sports may be problematic. The need to consider this issue is a key part of the restructuring approach to stress management interventions outlined in the following section. Specifically, sport psychologists may adopt a more individualized approach to the treatment of anxiety with the realization that advocating a general reduction or activation approach may not be appropriate for the demands of some sport tasks. The philosophy underpinning the restructuring approach suggests that rather than attempt to alter the level or amount of anxiety symptoms, it is more beneficial for practitioners to focus on the athletes' appraisals or interpretations of these symptoms. In particular, experiencing symptoms of competitive anxiety is considered a natural process in elite sport in which cognitive anxieties signify the importance of the event and help to stimulate the levels of effort needed to perform well, and somatic anxieties indicate a physical readiness to perform at a high level. Essentially, practitioners prescribe a range of psychological techniques that, when executed proficiently, allow performers to gain control over the anxiety symptoms, enabling the athletes to restructure and interpret anxiety (mental and physical) as helpful (or positive) for optimal performance. In this approach, practitioners essentially prescribe a psychological skills program that not only treats the competitive anxiety symptoms experienced by the performers, but also considers the activation demands of the tasks in their sport environment.

A restructuring approach to stress management intervention

The final remarks of the last section provide an applied rationale for adopting the restructuring approach in the development of stress management interventions for elite sport. It is also important, however, to provide a brief insight into the research that underpins the evidence base for the development of this approach. In addition to the applied reasoning, the restructuring approach has emerged as a direct consequence of developments in the research literature on competition stress, anxiety, and sport performance. Specifically, over the past 15 years, this research has consistently identified that certain athletes have the ability, or have learned over time, certain skills that enable them to interpret their anxiety symptoms as positive toward performance, whereas other athletes interpret their anxiety symptoms as negative. Studies have also suggested some important individual attributes that are related to the ability to interpret anxiety symptoms as positive toward performance. For example, athletes who view their competitive anxiety symptoms as more positive toward performance demonstrate better overall performance standards, are higher in skill level, feel more in control, exhibit higher levels of self-confidence, demonstrate a more resilient personality, and are more experienced and more highly competitive when compared to athletes who interpret

their anxiety symptoms as more negative toward performance. Given this association with positive performance and desirable personal qualities, applied researchers have sought to explore and identify the factors that enable athletes to achieve a positive interpretation of their competitive anxiety symptoms. This research has been undertaken with the explicit aim of informing the structure and content of possible stress management programs, and has helped construct the interventions used within the restructuring approach.

Recent studies with elite athletes have shown that elevated anxiety symptoms are not necessarily debilitative toward performance and therefore techniques designed to alter the levels of anxiety may not be appropriate for the activation demands of certain sports (e.g., weight lifting, explosive track events). Further, athletes with a positive interpretation of their anxiety symptoms have consistently suggested that it is the application of strategies that help them appraise their symptoms in a positive way that are most valuable to their performance preparation. The important psychological strategies involved in this approach are self-regulatory skills that provide athletes with a sense of perceived control over the environment and themselves, and enable them to maintain a high level of confidence that protects against negative anxiety interpretations. These strategies include cognitive restructuring and rationalization of anxiety symptoms (through the use of self-talk), goal setting practices that provide athletes with a level of control over the situation, and mental imagery that emphasizes control over their emotional state and depicts mastery of skills and performance. The following sections provide overviews of each of these psychological skills that indicate how they can be applied to help athletes foster more positive interpretations of anxiety symptoms.

Although essentially cognitive skills, the restructuring and rationalization of symptoms can be applied to help athletes cope with mental and physical anxiety. These skills are underpinned through the use of self-talk and are variations of approaches from cognitive rational-emotive behavioral therapy in the field of clinical psychology. Use of these skills is based on the premise that athletes experience and appraise situations that lead to beliefs that are either rational (i.e., positive interpretation of anxiety symptoms) or irrational (i.e., negative interpretation of anxiety symptoms). Rational beliefs lead to functional (beneficial) consequences for performance, whereas irrational beliefs lead to dysfunctional (harmful) consequences for performance. The application of these skills provides athletes with a framework to question the interpretation of the negative symptoms and turn them around to form a positive interpretation, thereby creating beliefs that lead to functional consequences for performance.

Traditionally, when learning the skills, athletes are taken through three progressive stages that focus on *identifying*, *disputing*, and then *replacing* their negative interpretations of anxiety symptoms. First, practitioners ask athletes to keep a diary of the negative mental and physical anxiety symptoms they experience. The athletes are then asked to *identify* that the symptoms are indeed irrational and will have a negative impact upon their preparation and performance. To achieve this, athletes apply the following questions to the symptoms they experience: "Is my appraisal based on fact?" "Does my appraisal help me achieve my sporting goals?," and "Does my appraisal help me to feel positive about my upcoming sport performance?" If the athletes answer "no" to these questions, then they are asked to question this initial appraisal and provide examples of how these interpretations can be *disputed*. An example of a thought process that would require disputing comes from the following extract from an interview with an elite field hockey player.

It is a combination of mental and physical things… they all come together, the worries make me stale, on the physical side I feel tense and in a rut. It becomes a completely negative thing and a completely negative feeling … I get anxious and worried and it is a distraction to me, a massive distraction.

This quote highlights the thought process that leads to a negative interpretation of pre-competition anxiety and a situation where experiencing these symptoms is viewed as harmful for their preparation and performance. Here, practitioners would educate

performers to *dispute* this irrational appraisal and *replace* it with a rationalized or *restructured* thought process, thereby creating a positive anxiety interpretation for performance. Continuing the example, the athletes would be educated to change the appraisal of their anxiety symptoms by questioning whether tension and worry are always detrimental to performance. The athletes would be asked to replace these thoughts with the ones suggesting that the worries they experience highlight the personal importance of the event and create an importance that equates to increased effort and a more focused and concentrated state. Finally, athletes are educated to consider that the physical symptoms they are experiencing actually indicate a level of physical preparedness for the task in hand and a readiness to physically perform optimally. Initially, the application of these skills can be challenging, and it is advised that athletes progress through the stages with a high degree of conscious thought and reliance on a suitably trained sport psychologist. Tapes, diaries, and scripts are often used to assist and educate the performer during this process to help create individualized restructuring programs. However, as athletes practice the skill and engage in ongoing dialog with the consultant, the application of the skill becomes a more automatic process. The following quote taken from an Olympic field hockey player provides a contextualized example of the restructuring and rationalization approach in action once the athlete has gained autonomy of the skill:

Nerves, anxiety and worry I can now actually turn them into a positive. If I am nervous and anxious I actually become more focused and it gives me a motivation to do it. It becomes a way of helping me, if I am anxious I feel focused and if I'm focused the nerves are helping me. So I think it is important for me to feel nervous and anxious, I can now turn it into giving me focus and it helps tell me there is a point behind why I am doing it (competing) and why I am feeling this way.

In an attempt to protect athletes from negative anxiety interpretations, goal setting and imagery skills can be used as confidence management strategies to help develop positive anxiety interpretations. Dealing with goal setting first, the notion of control as outlined earlier in this section becomes important. Specifically, in sport psychology, there are three main goal types: outcome, performance, and process goals. Outcome goals are based upon competitive outcomes (e.g., match result or position in a race) and typically involve some level of social comparison (i.e., the outcome is directly influenced by the performance of one's opponents). Performance goals are usually numerical and specify some form of absolute or self-referenced value (e.g., a split time in a 400-m race or a percentage successful pass completion rate in a team invasion game). Process goals focus on the demonstration of a certain behavior, skill, or strategy that relates to the sport task (e.g., maintaining a full follow through on a smash in badminton). Athletes maintain a greater degree of control over process and performance goals than outcome goals. The implication for this in relation to achieving a positive interpretation of anxiety is that when athletes maintain greater levels of control over a situation, they are more likely to interpret their anxiety symptoms as positive toward performance. Therefore, sport psychology consultants working toward positive anxiety interpretations should consider setting performance and process goal types as a protection mechanism. However, caution is advised here in relation to the idea that setting outcome goals is always a detrimental strategy for elite athletes. Although perceived controllability over outcome goals can be an issue, and unrealistic outcome goals can actually create anxiety for performers, the powerful motivational properties of outcome goals cannot be ignored. Therefore, athletes should set all the three types of goals, but place a greater degree of importance on performance and process goals as the competitive event becomes more imminent.

Mental imagery is a second psychological skill that athletes can use as a confidence management strategy to protect against negative interpretations of competitive anxiety. The functional classifications of imagery that have been most closely associated with attaining positive interpretations include athletes imaging the mastery of performance-related plans (e.g., tactical plans

being executed correctly), imaging the mastery of specific skills related to the athletes' role in competitive situations (e.g., successful shooting skills as a goal attack in netball) and imaging successfully managing the emotions that accompany competitive sport (e.g., imaging completion of a pre-shot routine that enables athletes to control their emotions and interpret anxiety symptoms as beneficial). As imagery is a notoriously difficult skill for athletes to master, sport psychologists usually work on performers' imagery skills using non-threatening scenarios before using imagery as a skill to restructure anxiety symptoms. The impact of any imagery intervention is partially dependent on the quality of the image the athlete can create with respect to submodalities of information. In this context, submodalities of information refers to the visual quality of the image (i.e., color and real-time movement), the auditory quality of the image (i.e., realistic crowd and background noise), kinesthetic properties of the image (i.e., associating the image with the feeling of real movements), and the perspectives (i.e., an internal perspective of viewing the image through one's own eyes or an external perspective as if viewing the image through a camera) from which athletes view the image. Specifically, the greater the control and vividness athletes possess over integrating these submodalities of information into their imagery drills (i.e., making their images as life-like as possible), the greater the impact the intervention has over the intended target. Hence, athletes could be asked to visualize a visit to shops, where the goals of the practice session would be to increase the visual quality of the images with a focus on seeing the images through an internal perspective with bright, vivid colors and movement that reflects the real-time action of the scene.

Once athletes have demonstrated a level of proficiency with the skill, practitioners target the imagery intervention toward maintaining confidence and creating a protection mechanism over negative anxiety interpretations. Initially, the sport psychologists and athletes produce a series of imagery scripts and audio tracks for the athletes to use to hone their imagery skills. For example, if the crux of the imagery routine that athletes require is a focus on images depicting mastery of certain skills within their sport, the sport psychologists ask the performers to (a) record the key skills for their role in their sport, for example, shooting skills as a goal attack in netball; (b) recount recent good performances of these skills, possibly making use of video; and (c) include as much information as possible to recreate a vivid image. The sport psychologists and athletes use this information to develop a series of imagery routines the athletes can use to create images depicting mastery of skills. The input of athletes into this process and the use of their knowledge base of the sport is a critical factor in creating tangible individualized imagery routines that have relevance to the performers. Scripts and recordings and one-to-one work with a sport psychologist underpins this work until the athletes become proficient at creating these images without the need for such tools. Sport psychologists use diary methods, checklists, and validated measures of imagery ability to consistently evaluate the athletes' progression with the learning of the skill. Once proficient at recreating sporting images in non-threatening situations away from the competitive arena, the athletes integrate the use of the skill into progressively increasing stressful environments within their sport (i.e., training, practice matches, main events) to gain full control over the skill in intense pressurized competitive settings.

A summary of the psychological skills presented under the umbrella of the restructuring approach is one that advocates combining various techniques into an integrated framework. Creating individualized psychological skills programs that are designed to meet the specific needs of the athlete is recommended. The important distinctions of these programs over those that attempt to solely manage the level of anxiety is the creation of an appraisal process whereby athletes gain control over themselves, the situation, and the anxiety symptoms that they experience in stressful environments. This approach also enables sport psychologists to take into account the specific activation demands of the tasks and events in which performers compete. A final caveat to the restructuring approach is that, to date, research has indicated that it is the more elite performers who may gain the most out of such an approach, whereas for lower level athletes, programs based on relaxation may be more suitable in the first instance. It appears, therefore, that the more advanced psychological skills used within the restructuring approach are more suited to elite level performers. Whichever approach is used, a suitably trained sport psychologist should design and deliver the content of the program, at least until athletes become proficient with the skills they are developing.

CASE STUDIES

Two case studies are presented to demonstrate approaches to treating competitive anxiety symptoms that athletes can experience. The reason for outlining two case studies is that although the restructuring approach provides a contemporary and complete treatment program for athletes, there are situations where the reduction approach is highly applicable. The decision of whether the sport psychologist uses the reduction approach or the restructuring approach should be based specifically on the activation levels required for optimal performance in the sport and the individual characteristics of the athlete. The two case studies presented here illustrate this point by featuring scenarios that feature Jon, an athlete in the sport of Olympic target rifle shooting, and Pete, an athlete in the sport of Olympic swimming.

CASE STUDY 1: JON

The athlete
Jon is a 34-year-old target rifle shooter who has been competing in his event for 10 years at a high standard.

Reason for consultancy
As a target rifle shooter, Jon had indicated to his coach and the sport psychologist for the team that he was having problems dealing with negative and distracting thoughts when preparing to shoot, and that he was experiencing high levels of physical tension in the shooting arm and shoulder prior to execution. He indicated to the consultant that he was feeling anxious prior to his events, that his performances were below par, and that he did not remember thinking or feeling this way when performing at his best.

Background
Following this discussion between Jon, the coach, and the sport psychologist, a consensus was reached that Jon would spend some time working with the sport psychologist to resolve the issue. In response to his concerns, the sport psychologist asked Jon to complete a series of validated questionnaires assessing his levels of anxiety and asked Jon to keep a diary of his thoughts and feelings prior to several important competitions.

CASE STUDIES (Continued)

Jon also sat down with the sport psychologist and discussed these issues in a one-to-one consultation. After triangulating this information, the sport psychologist established that Jon had high levels of both mental and physical anxieties both prior to performance and between shots on the rifle range.

Professional assessment

Given that the appropriate activation state that demonstrates a readiness to perform in target rifle shooting requires low levels of both mental and physical symptoms, the sport psychologist advocated an intervention program that followed the reduction approach to the treatment of competitive anxiety symptoms. As Jon indicated that his level of negative thoughts (i.e., cognitive anxiety) and negative feelings (i.e., somatic anxiety) were impairing his performance, and the evaluation indicated that both of these responses were high, the intervention targeted the reduction of both mental and physical anxiety symptoms.

Intervention

Jon was provided with an intervention program based on both mental and physical skills designed to reduce the levels of symptoms he experienced. As such, he was provided with a progressive muscle relaxation program to treat his physical anxieties, and was given a transcendental meditation program to help combat his mental anxieties. As Jon had indicated his symptoms were distracting him both prior to and during performance (i.e., between shots), both programs were designed as full progressive techniques in order for Jon to be able to use them before competing and between shots on the rifle range.

Outcome

Following the successful learning and application of the physical and mental relaxation programs prescribed by the sport psychologist (a process that spanned approximately 14 weeks), Jon indicated that he was able to effectively control his physical symptoms during competitive shooting performance. However, although the transcendental meditation program was having some success at reducing his mental anxieties, Jon still felt that this was a slight distraction to him. Following this concern, the sport psychologist advocated the use of a calming imagery technique. Following a further 5 weeks of training and learning this additional skill, Jon indicated he felt comfortable and able to regulate the levels of mental anxiety he experienced before and during shooting performance.

CASE STUDY 2: PETE

The athlete

Pete is a 27-year-old competitive 50 m freestyle swimmer. He has competed in his event for 9 years at the elite level and represented his country at one Olympic Games and one World Championship. Although he recently achieved the qualification time for the Olympic Games at his national trials, his time and performance in this race did not satisfy his, or his coaches', expectations.

Reason for consultancy

As a competitive 50 m freestyle swimmer, Pete had indicated to his national team's sport psychologist that prior to the recent Olympic trials and, indeed, during the warm up events to the trials, he was having problems dealing with distracting negative thoughts and high levels of muscle tension when in the waiting room preparing to race. Pete suggested that he was conscious of these mental and physical symptoms prior to the race and he felt they were having a negative impact on his pre-race preparation. He indicated that although he had experienced such symptoms all the way throughout his career, it was only recently that he felt unable to control their impact on him and how they were likely to affect his performance.

Professional assessment

Following this discussion, the sport psychologist and Pete agreed that they should put in place a program of work to alleviate the concerns Pete had expressed. Therefore, the sport psychologist asked Pete to complete a series of validated questionnaires assessing his pre-race anxiety levels and whether he viewed experiencing these symptoms as positive or negative toward his impending performance. The sport psychologist included information pertaining to how Pete was interpreting his anxiety-related symptoms due to the fact he had talked about a lack of control over how he thought the anxiety symptoms were likely to affect his future performance. The sport psychologist also consulted with Pete using an individual one-to-one approach to gain an understanding of his anxiety responses. Following this, the sport psychologist established that Pete's levels of pre-event anxiety were high and that he interpreted these symptoms as having a detrimental effect on his performance. Given that 50 m freestyle is an explosive event that requires a high degree of power as well as controlled aggression, the appropriate activation state for Pete that demonstrates a readiness to perform is one where he experiences a relatively high level of controlled physical and mental symptoms. In this instance, the sport psychologist advocated a treatment program that adhered to the principles of the restructuring approach. Prescribing techniques that only reduced Pete's symptoms could have had a detrimental effect on his performance, as he could have become too mentally and physically relaxed for the activation demands of this event, which, at Olympic level, typically lasts between 22 and 23 s.

Intervention program

Pete was provided with an intervention program based on restructuring the interpretation (negative to positive) of both his mental and physical anxieties. The main message of this program was to restructure Pete's anxiety interpretations to one where he viewed his mental symptoms as indicators of the importance of the event and his physical ones as indicators of his physical readiness to perform. The sport psychologist also provided some confidence maintenance techniques (i.e., goal setting and mental imagery) designed to help protect against potential negative interpretations of anxiety-related symptoms and any subsequent detrimental performance effects from the anxiety symptoms Pete experienced. As such, over time, Pete was tracked through the restructuring program outlined in this chapter. This process educated Pete to view his symptoms as a positive consequence for performance, removing the negative effects of anxiety on his race preparation.

Outcome

Following an intensive intervention program over a 10-week period, the treatment resulted in a reinterpretation of Pete's anxiety from negative to positive without reducing the level of anxiety symptoms (an indication of Pete attaining an appropriate activation state prior to competing). Indeed, following the intervention, Pete reported that he felt that his mental and physical symptoms were indicators of the importance of the event, how much effort he was prepared to invest in it, and how the symptoms could actually improve performance.

Further reading

Gould, D., Greenleaf, C., Krane, V. (2002) Arousal-anxiety and sport behavior. In T.S. Horn (ed.) *Advances in Sport Psychology*, 2nd Edn, pp. 207–241. Human Kinetics, Champaign, IL.

Hanton, S., Jones, G. (1999a) The acquisition and development of cognitive skills and strategies. I: Making the butterflies fly in formation. *The Sport Psychologist* **13**, 1–21.

Hanton, S., Jones, G. (1999b) The effects of a multimodal intervention on program performers. II: Training the butterflies to fly in formation. *The Sport Psychologist* **13**, 22–41.

Hardy, L., Jones, G., Gould, D. (1996) *Understanding Psychological Preparation for Sport: Theory and Practice of Elite Performance.* Wiley, Chichester, Sussex.

Jones, G. (1993) The role of performance profiling in cognitive behavioral interventions in sport. *The Sport Psychologist* **7**, 160–172.

Thomas, O., Maynard, I., Hanton, S. (2007) Intervening with athletes during the time leading up to competition: theory to practice II. *Journal of Applied Sport Psychology* **19**, 398–418.

Thomas, O., Mellalieu, S.D., Hanton, S. (in press) Stress management: recent directions in applied sport psychology research. *Advances in Applied Sport Psychology: A Review.* Routledge, London.

Chapter 5
Confidence in sport

Robin S. Vealey

Department of Kinesiology and Health, Miami University, Oxford, OH, USA

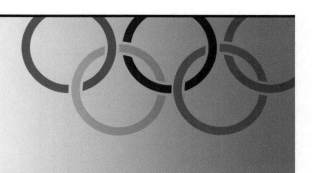

Introduction

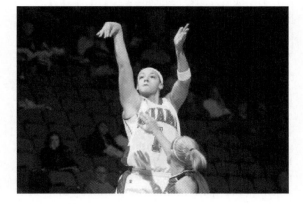

Confidence consistently appears as a key skill possessed by successful elite athletes, and international-level elite athletes have identified confidence as the most critical mental skill defining mental toughness. Knowing this, elite athletes have stated that the development and maintenance of confidence is one of their biggest needs in mental training. This is because along with its importance as a mental skill critical to sport performance, another defining characteristic of confidence is its fragility. Mia Hamm, all-time leading goal scorer in elite women's soccer, stated: "The thing about confidence I don't think people understand, is it's a day-to-day issue. It takes constant nurturing. It's not something you go in and turn on the light switch and say, 'I'm confident,' and it stays on until the light bulb burns out." Many athletes have admitted that confidence is a fragile psychological state. Indeed, fluctuations in confidence have been identified to account for differences in the best and worst performances in sport competition, and elite athletes have stated that the key to mental toughness is an "unshakable" self-confidence that is robust and resilient in the face of obstacles and setbacks.

The fact that confidence in sport is so important, and yet so fragile, makes it an intriguing topic in sport psychology. Most of the sport research on confidence has focused on *self*-confidence, or the belief that one has the internal resources, particularly abilities, to achieve success. Self-confidence is rooted in beliefs and expectations, and although there are multiple definitions of self-confidence, they all refer to *individuals' beliefs about their abilities and/or their expectations about achieving success based on these abilities*.

However, the self-confidence of athletes is embedded within increasingly broader layers of confidence (see Figure 5.1). For example, athletes understand that they have their own self-confidence and that their team has a collective level of confidence as well. One can have high self-confidence, but be part of a team with lower confidence. Many types of confidence shown in Figure 5.1 have been studied, and this multilevel view of confidence is important to consider in terms of its overall effect on athletes. Thus, it is important to have confidence in one's self, about fulfilling one's role within the team, in one's

Sport Psychology. 1st edition. Edited by Britton Brewer.
Published 2009 by Blackwell Publishing.
ISBN 978-1-4051-7363-6.

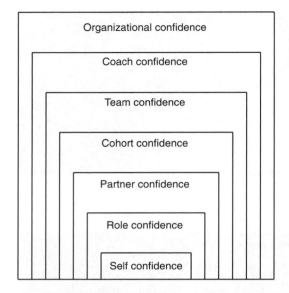

Figure 5.1. Multiple levels of confidence in sport

partner (e.g., pairs skating, beach volleyball), within one's cohort (e.g., ice hockey lines), one's team, one's coach, and one's organization (e.g., Olympic governing body). Highlighting the importance of having confidence in one's partner, which is crucial to the joint performance in many sports, a study of equestrian performance found that riders' self-confidence as well as riders' confidence *in their horses* were both significant predictors of dressage performance (and no, they didn't measure the horses' confidence!). Along with self-confidence, role, team, and coach confidence are examined in this chapter.

How is confidence measured in athletes?

Researchers often use psychological inventories to measure confidence in athletes, and there are several of these inventories available for research purposes. However, the best way for coaches and sport psychology consultants to assess confidence in athletes is through interpersonal discussion and observation of athletes' behavior. Following are some example questions that may help consultants understand factors related to athletes' confidence: "What are your thoughts, feelings, and actions that help you feel confident? What makes you feel

confident when training or competing in your sport? What are the thoughts, feelings, and actions that hurt your confidence in both training and competition? Where does your confidence come from or what is your confidence based on? When you lose focus or confidence or perform poorly, what strategies do you use to maintain or gain back confidence in yourself?"

Along with using questionnaires or interview questions, confidence can also be assessed in athletes using task-specific measures based on self-efficacy theory. As shown in Figure 5.2, athletes assess their confidence on varying levels of a specific task like basketball free throw shooting performance. Or, as shown in Figure 5.3, a hierarchy of performance levels against which to judge self-confidence in pitching a curveball in softball can be used with athletes. Yet another way to measure self-confidence in athletes is to use a non-hierarchical measure, which is simply a list of skills that athletes use to rate their perceived ability to perform successfully. For example, wrestlers would rate their abilities to successfully perform an escape, get reversal, get takedown by throw, ride opponent, and so forth. Therefore, confidence can be assessed by putting together an appropriate measure of challenges and skills associated with successful performance in specific sports.

Interview questions or task-specific measures can be used to assess the various types of confidence shown in Figure 5.1. Along with understanding athletes' personal confidence, questions could also be posed to assess their confidence in their ability to fulfill their role on the team, in key teammates, in the team as a whole, in their coach, and even in their organization.

What do athletes need to be confident about?

Athletes have identified several important types of confidence including the need to believe in their abilities to execute physical skills, attain high levels of physical fitness, make correct decisions, execute mental skills such as focusing attention and managing nervousness, bounce back from

How certain are you that you can successfully shoot a basketball from the free throw line?

	0%	10%	20%	30%	40%	50%	60%	70%	80%	90%	100%
10 out of 100											
20 out of 100											
30 out of 100											
40 out of 100											
50 out of 100											
60 out of 100											
70 out of 100											
80 out of 100											
90 out of 100											
100 out of 100											

Figure 5.2. Hierarchical measure of level and strength of free throw shooting confidence

How certain are you that you can throw a curve ball for a strike...

1. In practice?
2. When warming up before the game?
3. In early innings with no score and no runners on base?
4. In early innings with runners on base?
5. In middle innings with the scored tied and runners on base?
6. In late innings with the score tied?
7. In late innings with the score tied and runners on base?
8. In the final inning with a one run lead and runners on base?
9. In the final inning with a one run lead, two outs, full count, and bases loaded?

Figure 5.3. Performance levels to judge confidence in softball pitching

mistakes, overcome obstacles and setbacks, achieve mastery and personal performance standards, and win and demonstrate superiority over opponents. Figure 5.4 offers a categorization of these various types of confidence identified by athletes as important in sport. Athletes should develop and maintain beliefs about their abilities to (a) win (outcome self-confidence), (b) perform successfully in relation to certain standards (performance self-confidence), (c) self-regulate to manage their thoughts and emotions as well as bounce back in demonstrating resilience (self-regulatory self-confidence), and (d) execute the physical skills, achieve fitness/ training levels, and learn new skills needed to be successful in their sports (physical self-confidence).

Influence of self-confidence on athletes' performance

A great deal of research in sport psychology has examined the influence of self-confidence on athletes' performance. This research has ranged from

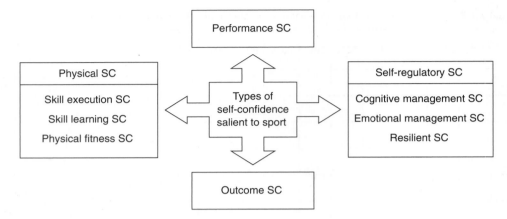

Figure 5.4. Types of self-confidence needed by athletes in sport

experimental studies to field research to qualitative interviews with athletes about the importance of confidence.

Experimental studies

Beginning in the 1970s, a line of experimental research studies using non-athletes as research participants investigated the influence of self-confidence on motor performance. Many of these studies used anxiety-inducing tasks such as back dives to examine avoidance behavior. This research showed that confidence enhanced performance. Another group of experimental studies manipulated research participants' confidence using deception to see how confidence influenced performance. In all instances, participants manipulated to have high self-confidence (e.g., being told they were competing against an injured opponent) outperformed participants who were manipulated to have low self-confidence. Other experimental research showed that "cognitive psyching" by using self-confidence exhortations to oneself increased strength performance as compared to a control group who did not psych themselves up.

Confidence studied in natural competitive sport settings

Most of the research since the mid-1980s has examined the relationship between self-confidence and performance with athletes in natural competitive settings. Through advanced statistical techniques

such as meta-analyses, in which many studies are statistically aggregated to make broad conclusions about a research area, self-confidence has been shown to have a positive, yet moderate, relationship with performance. An important finding has been that self-confidence assessed *after* performance is more strongly related to performance than confidence assessed *prior to* performance, suggesting that prior performance influences confidence more strongly than confidence influences performance.

Descriptive studies of confidence in athletes

International-level elite athletes have identified self-confidence as the most critical mental skill defining mental toughness; and in interviews with Olympic champions, their coaches, and parents or significant others, self-confidence has been identified as a key mental skill to successful performance at the elite level. Olympic coaches have identified self-confidence as a very important influence on their athletes' performance. Also, self-confidence has differentiated successful and less successful athletes at the elite level.

How does confidence influence athletes' performance?

A key question is *how* self-confidence works to influence the way that athletes perform. Self-confidence can be thought of as the "mental modifier," because confidence seems to modify how athletes feel about, respond to, and think about everything that happens to them in sport. For example, self-confidence has been shown to positively predict athletes' effort and persistence in sport. An elite athlete explained how confidence increases effort: "When I feel confident, it just drives me on more and makes me try harder, raises my game and the intensity of my effort and preparation" (Hanton et al., 2004). Confidence also affects the choices that athletes make about joining and continuing participation in sport. For example, youth wrestlers who have remained in the sport have reported higher self-confidence than wrestlers who have dropped out, and runners with higher self-confidence have chosen more difficult tasks than those with less self-confidence.

Confident athletes have been shown to *think better* than less-confident athletes. Confident athletes cope better, make more productive causal attributions (i.e., reasons they use to explain why they succeed and fail), set more challenging goals, and are more motivated than less-confident athletes. Self-confidence is also related to effective concentration and decision-making.

Interestingly, self-confidence is critical in buffering the negative effects of anxiety on athletes' performance. Self-confidence seems to buffer the effects of anxiety on athletes' performance by allowing them to tolerate higher levels of anxiety before experiencing decrements in performance. If athletes feel confident and in control, they maintain positive expectancies of goal attainment and coping abilities, and respond in anxious situations with increased effort, persistence, and performance. However, for athletes who doubt their ability to cope and succeed, anxiety is debilitating because they withdraw efforts based on their beliefs that they cannot control themselves or their environments. These findings emphasize the important point that self-confidence is not the absence of anxiety, but rather a facilitative quality that enables athletes to engage in self-regulatory responses (e.g., reframing, effort, coping) to manage their anxiety in productive ways and perform effectively. This is best explained by an elite gymnast, who stated: "... I had doubts, that everyone has, like what happens if I fall off again ... but I

mean that's only momentarily and then you start telling yourself just to calm down and get back on and do it cleanly ... I knew I could do it easily ... But ... I was confident that ... I could do it – and, it's just [that] your heart rate goes up and you feel your chest pounding" (Edwards et al., 2002).

What are important sources of confidence for athletes?

The most important source of confidence for athletes is performance success. This has been found with youth, high school, collegiate, elite, and master athletes. The importance of performance success in developing confidence is aptly described by a member of the US Women's Ice Hockey team who won the gold medal in the 1998 Olympic Games: "... having played Canada 15 times was a huge factor, because they went from having this kind of aura about them, of being ... the best team, and after you play them several times, you're 'hey, they are just another team, and we [just] as good,' ... with each win that we had against Canada, and even each loss, because it was a one-goal loss ... or it was a really close game ... so each victory or each close loss kind of built that confidence up ..." (Haberl & Zaichkowsky, 1999). This quote emphasizes that even the objective outcome of losing can serve as a successful performance experience for the enhancement of confidence if athletes perceive that they performed well and gained insights from the experience.

Other sources of confidence important to athletes include training and preparation, modeling, leadership, and social influences. Athletes cite both physical and mental preparation as critical to their confidence, and coaches tend to use instruction and drilling in practice to build confidence in their athletes. Mental training techniques such as imagery and self-talk have been shown to enhance confidence. Confidence can be enhanced by watching another person performing a skill (modeling), particularly if the model is similar to the athletes themselves or if the model is highly skilled. Similarly, coaches who serve as effective models and/or leaders are important sources of confidence. Typically, multiple sources are used to build confidence. For example, positive feedback is a strong source of confidence when it is provided after performance success, but considerably weaker as a source by itself. Coaches can demonstrate effective leadership skills and verbally persuade their athletes that they can perform skills successfully. An elite athlete explained: "Being verbally persuaded by your coach is the best protection against any worries or concerns. It's linked to your confidence … you don't think negative when you've got positive thoughts in your mind and your coach is saying to you that you are going to do it. You know it's going to be a … good performance" (Hanton et al., 2004).

Differences in confidence based on gender and skill

Confidence differences between males and females are related to the perceived gender appropriateness of the task being performed. Females have shown lower self-confidence on "gender-inappropriate" activities, but no gender differences in confidence have emerged for performance on gender-neutral activities. Research has demonstrated that the more "masculine" an activity is considered, the greater are the differences in self-confidence between males and females. Sex-typing works both ways, as males have shown higher confidence on "male" tasks and females have shown higher confidence on "female" tasks.

Gender differences have also been found in the sources of confidence identified by athletes. Demonstrating ability in relation to others and winning are important antecedents of male athletes' confidence, whereas personal goals/standards and social support from coaches and teammates are important antecedents of female athletes' confidence. A robust finding in the literature is that advanced, elite, expert athletes have higher levels of self-confidence than beginner, non-elite, non-expert athletes, irrespective of gender.

Confidence in coaches

The study of self-confidence in sport has progressed to focus on confidence in coaches as well as athletes.

The importance of self-confidence for coaches is apparent in the following quotes from inexperienced coaches: "I wasn't as confident as I wished I had been from the start … and I think that weakened the power of my coaching." "I should have started out just being more confident in myself. If I had been a little stronger, I would have been more effective throughout the season" (Weiss et al., 1991).

Coaches' confidence has been predicted by prior success, coaching experience, perceived athlete talent, and social support. Similar to findings with athletes, social support is a stronger source of confidence for female coaches than for male coaches. In structured interviews, coaches have identified the development of their athletes, their own coaching education and development, knowledge and preparation, leadership skills, athlete support, and experience as sources for their coaching confidence. Coaches who are highly confident that their teams will perform well have tended to attribute that confidence to good competitive and practice performance, preparation, favorable social comparison with the opponent, and a belief in their team's resilience. In contrast, coaches who are less confident that their teams will perform well have tended to attribute that confidence to unfavorable social comparison with the opponent, bad competitive and practice performance, inconsistency in the team's performance, physical problems, and low athlete self-confidence. Coaches identify performance success, preparation, and social support as important sources of confidence.

As shown in Figure 5.5, coaching confidence affects coaches' own behaviors and self-perceptions, as well as the behaviors, self-perceptions, and affective responses of athletes on the team. Research has shown that high-confident coaches provide more praise and encouragement to athletes than low-confident coaches, whereas low-confident coaches perform more instructional and organizational behaviors than high-confident coaches.

With regard to performance, high-confident coaches have higher winning percentages than low-confident coaches, and coaching confidence is predictive of team performance. Coaching confidence has also been positively associated with team confidence, but not individual athlete self-confidence. With regard to gender differences,

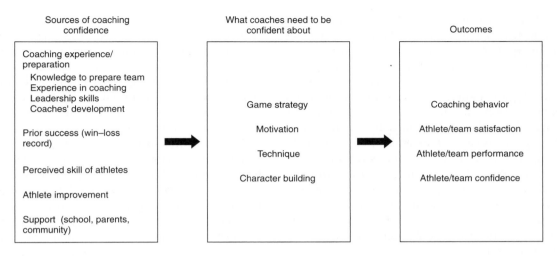

Figure 5.5. Model of coaching confidence

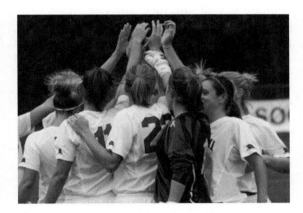

coaching confidence has been found to be no different between male and female head coaches.

Role and team confidence

As discussed earlier, the study of self-confidence has evolved to focus on confidence beyond the "self." Role confidence has been conceptualized as athletes' perceived capabilities to successfully perform in interdependent ways within their roles on teams. In a study of basketball players, starters reported greater role confidence than non-starters, although there were no differences in self-efficacy between the two groups. After controlling for self-efficacy, role efficacy was significantly related to athletes' performance as assessed by teammates and coaches.

Team confidence is the team's shared belief in their collective abilities to successfully perform. Because of the required task interdependence and the close interpersonal relations evident within sport teams, team confidence is a better predictor of team performance than aggregates of team members' confidence. In one study, individual self-confidence was the strongest predictor of personal perceptions of team confidence in the sport of rowing, which requires almost perfect synchronicity among teammates. That is, rowers who were more confident in their own abilities to row were more likely to feel confident about their crew's abilities to row.

Interventions to enhance confidence in athletes

Athletes who use the mental training techniques of relaxation, self-talk, and goal setting extensively have higher levels of self-confidence prior to competition than athletes who use these techniques less frequently. Self-confidence can be increased through mental training interventions using imagery, self-talk, goal setting, and relaxation training. Self-confidence can also be facilitated by numerous multimodal interventions, which use a combination of mental training strategies and techniques to enhance self-confidence. The integration of mental and physical training is a powerful achievement approach to enhancing confidence in athletes.

As an example of an empirically validated intervention to enhance confidence in athletes, goals, imagery, and self-talk were incorporated into personalized pre-competitive and pre-race routines to enhance self-confidence in competitive swimmers. The swimmers were taught how to identify and focus on intrapersonal goals within their control, such as performance times and race processes. Written scripts and audiotapes were developed for each of the swimmers so they could rehearse their typical thoughts and feelings experienced before a competitive race, along with a rationalizing and reframing strategy in which their thoughts and feelings were viewed as natural and potential facilitators of performance. The swimmers also mentally rehearsed their controllable race processes, and practiced these mental exercises three times each week. In addition, pre-race routines were developed in which each swimmer visually recalled positive training and competitive experiences, focused on process goals for the upcoming race, and read cue cards with self-affirmation statements to accept and use their feelings of nervousness. All intervention swimmers increased their post-intervention confidence scores, whereas the control swimmer did not.

Another example of an effective intervention to enhance confidence in athletes was a season-long (25 weeks) mental training program with junior elite tennis players. The mental training program consisted of goal setting, positive self-talk, concentration routines, arousal regulation techniques, and imagery. Athletes were directed in setting physical, conditioning, and mental performance goals, and they continuously charted their progress and made revisions across the season. They learned the basic principles of productive self-talk by identifying their negative thoughts, developing a trigger to refocus their thoughts more productively, and practicing positive body language. They worked on identifying their optimal arousal levels, and learned relaxation and activation techniques (e.g., centering, progressive muscle relaxation, physical drills to increase arousal) that they could use to optimize arousal into their preferred zones. They developed personal routines to be used between points in their matches, and mentally rehearsed perfect technique on various shots and successful match tactics. All of the participants in the intervention group increased their confidence and tennis performance after the mental training program.

Overall, the research supports the effectiveness of mental training on the enhancement of self-confidence in athletes. The various mental training techniques, such as imagery, goal setting, self-talk, and relaxation, can be combined in different ways, used in conjunction with physical training, and specifically tailored to enable athletes to feel more confident, energized, and focused.

CASE STUDY: An Intervention to Enhance Confidence

Athlete
Brooke is the starting point guard for her country's national basketball team.

Reason for consultancy
In a game a few months prior to the Olympic Games, Brooke missed two free throws in the closing seconds of a game that would have allowed her team to win. Immediately after that experience, Brooke's confidence at the free throw line plummeted and her shooting percentage dropped from 87% to 50%. With the Games coming up in a few months, the coaches

were concerned and told Brooke that she may lose her starting position because the point guard must be able to make free throws in the closing minutes of tight games. Brooke then put additional pressure on herself and her shooting slump worsened.

Professional assessment
In talking with Brooke, it became apparent that she had fixated on the key missed free throws when her team lost. Her images and self-talk had become negative and less controllable, and her

attentional focus at the line was inward as she was paralyzed into controlled processing (thinking about how to shoot) as opposed to allowing her shot to flow freely through automatic processing. She had lost her belief in herself to make free throws, particularly in critical situations.

Intervention

Confidence is a difficult skill to mend, because its main source is performance success. Thus, an intervention to enhance confidence should combine a progressive physical training strategy with a mental training strategy that attempts to redirect an athletes' focus, self-talk, and personal images. Because Brooke lost confidence in her free throw shot, she agreed to change her pre-shot routine to wipe away the negative memory and triggers that reminded her of the missed free throws. This change in routine was early enough prior to the Games to become habitual and familiar to Brooke, and she liked the new yet comfortable pre-shot approach. She described it as a feeling that she had left the old free throw "problem" behind by changing her routine.

To create this new routine, Brooke engaged in a "centering" exercise where she carefully considered how she wanted to physically feel as well as what she wanted to think about when she got to the free throw line. She decided to engage the feeling of being strong in her legs and balanced at the line. She would take her stance carefully and flex her knees a few times to cue the strong and balanced feeling. Her attentional focus was a smooth uncoiling of her body and the ball floating softly over the front of the rim. Her self-talk mantra was "strong, smooth, soft" which verbally and visually led her through the steps of her routine.

Once her routine was created, she began practicing it in sets of 10 repetitions at 5 ft, 10 ft, and then 15 ft (the free throw line) in front of the basket. This gave her a progression to follow, with the intent of practicing the routine enough to make it automatic and useful. And prior to physically practicing at each station, she mentally practiced her new routine and shooting the 10 repetitions at each spot. As time progressed in training sessions with the team, the coaches eased Brooke back into pressure situations by having her shoot free throws with consequences (e.g., running sprints) if she missed. This allowed her to practice her new routine in simulated competitive situations.

Outcome

The routine was developed to occupy Brooke's mind when she went to the free throw line. Instead of telling athletes "don't think," it is better to help them develop a plan for how to think when negative thinking becomes a problem. Brooke really liked "shedding" the old routine and leaving her problem behind her, and the fresh start and mental plan coupled with systematic physical practice allowed her to overcome her "choking" response at the line. She did come back and ask for one more adjustment. Her routine at the line was working, but she felt uncontrollable at the initial moment when she was fouled and realized that she was going to the line. She said she would have a quick "Oh, no" moment where she felt fear about going to the line. Through discussion, the first thing Brooke was made to realize and accept was that fear is okay and normal in that situation. She learned a response plan for the moment she was fouled, in which she could acknowledge her fear but also her confidence that she would make the shot. She chose to focus her attention immediately on how prepared she was to shoot the free throw by saying to herself, "I'm ready, I'm strong, I'm smooth." She worked on physically portraying confidence in her posture and walk to the line, and visually rehearsed the thoughts, feelings, and posture she would engage in prior to shooting. In time, Brooke lost the fear feeling, but continued using her strategies in thinking a specific way in walking to the line as well as engaging her very specific pre-shot routine. Mental training didn't make Brooke infallible—she occasionally missed free throws—but this was infrequent in occurrence and was not the result of choking or loss of confidence. Brooke learned to trust her preparation and follow her mental plan, and was able to do that because she spent extra time physically practicing free throws. She came to understand that the mental training allowed her to physically train in more effective ways, which allowed her to enjoy more success in basketball.

References

Edwards, T., Kingston, K, Hardy, L., Gould, D. (2002) A qualitative analysis of catastrophic performances and the associated thoughts, feelings, and emotions. *The Sport Psychologist* **16**, 1–19.

Haberl, P., Zaichkowsky, L. (1999) The U.S. women's Olympic gold medal ice hockey team: optimal use of sport psychology for developing confidence. In R. Lidor & K.P. Henschen (eds.) *The Psychology of Team Sports*, pp. 217–233. Fitness Information Technology, Morgantown.

Hanton, S., Mellalieu, S.D., Hall, R. (2004) Self-confidence and anxiety interpretation: qualitative investigation. *Psychology of Sport and Exercise* **5**, 477–495.

Weiss, M.R., Barber, H., Sisley, B.L., Ebbeck, V. (1991) Developing competence and confidence in novice female coaches: II. Perceptions of ability and affective experiences following a season-long coaching internship. *Journal of Sport and Exercise Psychology* **13**, 336–362.

Further reading

Feltz, D.L., Short, S.E., Sullivan, P.J. (2008) *Self-Efficacy in Sport*. Human Kinetics, Champaign.

Vealey, R.S. (2005) *Coaching for the Inner Edge*. Fitness Information Technology, Morgantown.

Vealey, R.S., Chase, M.A. (2008) Self-confidence in sport. In T.S. Horn (ed.) *Advances in Sport Psychology*, 3rd Edn, pp. 65–97. Human Kinetics, Champaign.

Chapter 6
Mental preparation for training and competition

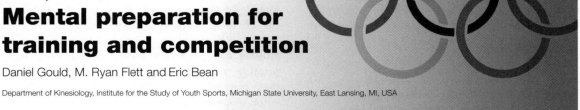

Daniel Gould, M. Ryan Flett and Eric Bean

Department of Kinesiology, Institute for the Study of Youth Sports, Michigan State University, East Lansing, MI, USA

I prepare mentally each and every day… I have a lot of mental exercises that I use in preparation for any large event.
　　　　　—Olympic Athlete (Greenleaf et al., 2001).

Make a list — an in-list and an out-list — of things that are necessary. List things that will help you and hurt you in trying to win the gold. If the issue will help you win the gold, write it on the list. If it's something that will hurt your performance, throw it in the trash basket, and deal with it after the Olympics.
　　　　　—Olympic Gold Medalist (Gould et al., 1999).

More than anything athletes need to have a routine established and they need to stick with that routine and take refuge in that routine, because at the Games everything changes.
　　　　　—Olympic Athlete (Greenleaf et al., 2001).

Athletes and coaches constantly talk about mental preparation, psyching up, getting their game face on, and getting emotionally prepared to perform. Discussed less often, but of equal importance, is mental preparation for practices. In fact, recent research has shown that top athletes and coaches not only focus on the best ways to mentally ready themselves for competitions, but also for routine training sessions. Given the emphasis athletes and coaches place on mental preparation, it is not surprising that sport psychology researchers have been highly interested in the topic. Their research has shown that mental preparation is critical for sport success for both individual athletes and teams.

Sport Psychology. 1st edition. Edited by Britton Brewer.
Published 2009 by Blackwell Publishing.
ISBN 978-1-4051-7363-6.

Although mental preparation is often discussed by athletes and coaches as being critically important, optimal strategies for mental preparation are typically left to trial and error learning. However, with the growth and acceptance of applied sport psychology, more emphasis is being placed on purposefully instructing athletes and teams on optimal ways to mentally prepare. This chapter is designed to summarize what is known about effective mental preparation for athletes and teams. Guidelines for effective mental preparation are also forwarded. The chapter concludes with a series of case studies demonstrating how individual athletes and teams mentally prepare for peak performance in both training and competition.

What is mental preparation?

Although coaches and athletes often refer to the importance of mental preparation, they seldom define it precisely. This is problematic, as the concept can be viewed in many ways. For example, mental preparation can be considered very broadly as anything athletes do to ready themselves for sport involvement or in a very specific manner as the techniques a basketball player uses to ready himself or herself for a particular free throw. For the purpose of this chapter, mental preparation is defined as those cognitive, emotional, and behavioral strategies athletes and teams use to arrive at an ideal performance state or condition that is related to optimal psychological states and peak performance for either competition or practice. Discussion of mental preparation is also limited to purposeful efforts that athletes and coaches use to ready themselves, although it is recognized that many athletes may unknowingly engage in certain preparatory behaviors through force of habit or because those in their sport have always done it that way.

What research and practice say about effective mental preparation

Over the last 30 years, research in sport psychology has repeatedly shown that an athlete's mentality influences his or her performance. The earliest research was conducted in laboratory settings or controlled field environments and involved athletes mentally preparing or psyching up in a particular manner (e.g., trying to narrow their focus, arouse themselves, use imagery) for a predetermined time and then performing different motor tasks. Results revealed that mental preparation did indeed influence performance (when compared to participants who did not mentally prepare). However, none of the mental preparation techniques was consistently superior. In contrast, the most effective type of mental preparation depended on the type of task being performed (e.g., strength versus fine motor accuracy tasks). This implies that athletes must mentally prepare themselves differently depending on the type of task being performed.

In a similar but separate line of research, Russian-born sport psychologist Yuri Hanin has conducted research for several decades aimed at identifying athletes' individualized zones of optimal functioning (IZOF). Hanin's research has shown that athletes have certain idiosyncratic patterns of emotions that are associated with best performance. When they experience these emotions within an optimal range, superior performance results. However, when athletes or teams are out of their zone of optimal functioning, subpar performance results. The "zone" is like an *emotional recipe* in that there are several emotional ingredients in an individual's zone—not just one emotion—and these emotions interact to determine one's ability to mobilize and to control energy.

An athlete's optimal zone of functioning is important because it identifies the psychological state that one needs to achieve best performance—and contrasts this zone with the psychological state associated with worst performance. In addition to looking at the recipe (i.e., the types of emotions), the intensity of these feelings should also be considered. Emotional intensity can be presented to athletes metaphorically, as an optimal body temperature. Athletes function best when they are at their optimal body temperature (or, in this case, emotional temperature). Inferior performance results when they are below or above their optimal temperature (they are cold or have a fever). Extending this notion, mental preparation is akin to a thermostat, where athletes can do specific things—like listening to certain types of music or thinking of motivational phrases—to increase their emotional activation level as needed (when below their optimal target zone). Athletes can also use stress management and other coping techniques to cool off when their emotional level is too hot. Mental preparation, then, helps athletes develop cognitive, emotional, and behavioral strategies that can be used to regulate their emotional and cognitive state in the direction of their zone of optimal functioning.

As illustrated by the field hockey player's IZOF that is shown in Figure 6.1, "Anna" plays best when she is aggressively calm (i.e., moderately aggressive and moderately-to-very calm). She does not want to be panicky-aggressive or sluggishly calm. Confidence is even more important for Anna. Her optimal level of confidence should be between six and eight (on a 10-point thermostat). Anna does not want to be too confident, but her zone of *worst* functioning is very close to her *optimal* zone, so this is a very important variable for her to manage before and during competition. When Anna is mentally calm, her attitude is moderately aggressive, and she is confident, the rest of her profile normally falls into the optimal zone. Preparation and coping strategies will help her to control these three factors, making her performance more focused and energized.

Key mental preparation principles

With this theoretical orientation as a base, the remainder of this chapter focuses on what has been

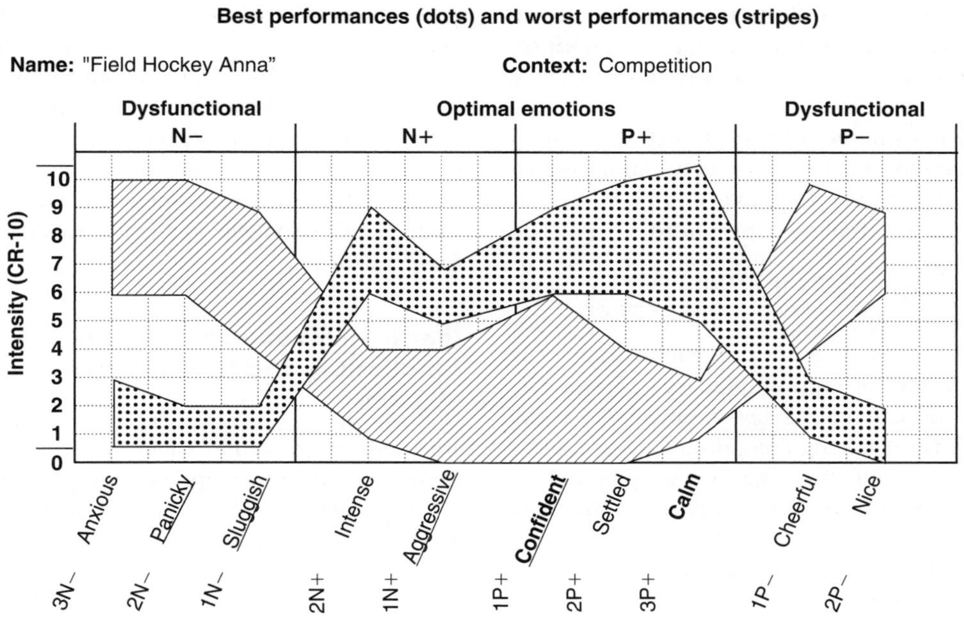

Best performances (dots) and worst performances (stripes)

Figure 6.1. Example of an athlete's individualized zones of optimal functioning. The figure is organized into four columns, representing combinations of (N) negative, (P) positive, (+) helpful, and (−) harmful emotions. The optimal profile generally shows an iceberg, or inverted-U, profile. The zone for worst performance is typically U-shaped

learned about mental preparation. Key findings are summarized in the following section.

Mental preparation counts

Sport psychology researchers have been interested in how athletes' psychological factors and characteristics influence performance. From this research, it is clear that psychological characteristics differ between more and less effective athletes and teams. Moreover, the ability to mentally prepare is considered a key component of such differences. Research with Olympic athletes and teams has consistently shown that more successful athletes spend more time on their mental preparation than their less successful counterparts.

Mental preparation for practice is critical

When most people think about mental preparation, their first thoughts are of psychological

techniques that athletes and teams use to ready themselves for competition. However, recent sport psychology research has shown that mental preparation is not only critical for competitive performance, but is equally important for training. For example, in a recent study of world and Olympic champion athletes and their coaches and sport psychologists, views of mental toughness were solicited. It was found that attitudes and beliefs about training were viewed as key elements of mental toughness. In particular, it was stated that mentally tough athletes keep motivation levels high for training by using long-term goals as a source of motivation while at the same time exhibiting the patience, discipline, and self-control to realistically work toward long-term objectives. Mentally tough performers were also seen as gaining as much control as possible over their training and using every aspect of the training environment to their advantage. Finally, they were perceived as being very competitive in practice and pushing themselves to reach their potential in training. When coupled with other research, these findings clearly suggest that considerable attention should be paid to mentally preparing for practice and training sessions.

There are a number of ways athletes can mentally prepare for practice. First, they can develop a set ritual or routine for approaching practices. For example, as an athlete changes into his practice attire, he can take a deep breath and park his off-the-field thoughts in his locker as he hangs up his street clothes. Then, as he walks to the practice field, he can think about one thing he wants to focus on or accomplish during practice. During the warm-up, he can take a few moments to focus his thoughts on having a good practice and visualize doing so. Finally, as he finishes practice, he may take a few moments to think about the most important things he learned that day and later record the lessons learned from the session into his training journal.

Another way to mentally prepare for practice is to field-test one's competition mental preparation approach. For example, a figure skater may approach an upcoming practice where judges will be present by treating it as a run-through of her competition day. She might eat a pregame meal at the appropriate time, arrive at the rink at her preferred time, warm up in her desired way, and then perform her long program with no stopping regardless of whether errors occur. Of course, practicing one's approach to competition would only be done from time to time and not on a daily basis.

The practice environment also offers numerous opportunities to develop emotional management skills that will not only help to make practices more productive, but will also allow athletes to have mental preparation skills that can be used in competitions. For instance, by its very nature, practice has numerous failures and mistakes built into it. An athlete can use these challenges to develop and practice refocusing strategies when frustrated by making mistakes (e.g., take a deep breath and visualize flushing the mistake out of the system, stop negative thoughts, and replace them with more positive ones). In addition to being challenging, most sports practice more than they compete. As such, practice and training provide more opportunities for players to refine coping strategies

to overcome arousal, frustration, fatigue (flatness), and other adverse mental conditions. Over time and through practice, these coping strategies will become more effective. It is also important for athletes to sometimes modify the strategies they use in practice to meet the unique demands of competition. Whether such adjustments are small or large, using practices to develop mental skills is beneficial for competition.

Identifying zones of optimal functioning and how to arrive at them

Top performers learn to identify what emotions make up their zone of optimal functioning and the levels of those emotions needed for best practices and performances. This can be accomplished by reflecting on the previous best and worst performances. Keeping a journal of competitive experiences can also help to develop or edit one's optimal recipe. It also helps athletes to be more self-aware. It is important to note that zones of optimal functioning need not be overly complex or analytical. Many athletes simply recognize the general feeling state they need to perform best, along with a few key emotions associated with that state they. This state can be summarized with a few cue/trigger words. They also learn self-regulation strategies to mentally prepare and, in so doing, manage their emotions so that they get to and remain in their zone of optimal functioning. Lastly, they develop refocusing strategies to deal with unexpected events that can occur before and during competition. It is imperative, then, that aspiring athletes learn to identify their IZOF and psychological strategies for getting into the zone by following the strategies discussed in this chapter.

Mental preparation routines need to enhance self-confidence

One of the most robust findings in the sport psychology literature is that more successful performers consistently differ from their less successful counterparts in their self-confidence or self-efficacy. Simply put, they believe they can execute the skills and muster the persistence needed to achieve top performance and cope with any adversity that arises. Confidence, however, is not just thinking positively. Rather, it is an inner belief most often based on past performance accomplishments and the achievement of goals, while at the same time being influenced by a variety of additional sources. It is crucial that athletes' mental preparation enhances their confidence (e.g., keep themselves relaxed so feelings of anxiety don't trigger negative thoughts and self-doubt, remind themselves of previous performance accomplishments, execute certain physical skills in a prescribed fashion). In fact, having a consistent mental preparation routine is an important source of confidence for many athletes because familiarity and certainty have been shown to enhance confidence, whereas uncertainty lessens it.

The role of confidence is just as important in teams. Research shows that team confidence is related to performance. Moreover, when it comes to team confidence, it could be said that the whole is greater than the sum of the parts. Team confidence has not been found to simply be the additive effect of individual athlete confidence levels, it is more than that. Team confidence involves trust and confidence in one's teammates and coaches, as well as the individual athlete's confidence in themselves. Team confidence, then, is much more than the sum of each individual's self-confidence.

Prioritization and goal setting

Setting and prioritizing appropriate goals are important components of mental preparation. Goal setting helps athletes direct their attention to important elements of the task, is associated with enhanced motivation, and affects psychological states like self-confidence and anxiety. However, it is also clear that not all goals are equally effective in enhancing performance. For example, goals should be difficult but realistic, specific, and tied to specific goal achievement strategies. In terms of mental preparation, a key difference between more versus less successful competitors is the fact that more successful athletes set specific goals for practice, not just competition. In the competitive preperformance venue, most top competitors focus on both

process (e.g., a downhill skier focusing on keeping his arms out in front of him and letting his outside ski run) and performance goals (e.g., a 10,000 m runner trying to run specific split times) versus focusing sole attention on outcome goals (e.g., beating an opponent). It is not that top competitors do not want to win. In contrast, they are very competitive and want to win very badly. However, they find that at or during competition it is most effective to focus on performance and process goals as these are much more under their personal control. They want to win, so they focus on *how to* win.

The importance of developing performance routines

More versus less effective performers have specific physical and mental routines that they adhere to prior to and during competition. For example, successful figure skaters prepare the same way for each of their competitions. They won't mentally prepare differently for the more important competitions or do less for competitions that are of lesser importance. In contrast, less successful athletes tend to psych up more, change their precompetitive routines, or fail to adhere to their routines in pressure situations. A key to optimal mental preparation, then, is to develop and adhere to consistent precompetitive mental preparation routines.

Because things do not always go as planned, top performers must also learn to adapt their normal mental preparation routines. For example, a swimmer may have a mental preparation routine that she executes 30–40 min prior to her race. Knowing this, she always tries to arrive at the venue in plenty of time to execute her preparation routine. However, she also realizes that on some occasions things do not go as planned (e.g., the bus gets delayed in traffic and the team arrives late to the pool), and she will need to have a shortened version of her routine developed and practiced so that she can execute it in 5–10 min. Similarly, at other times events will be delayed and she will have longer time than expected to mentally ready herself. She must be prepared to hold her focus over a longer length of time. These variations of the normal mental preparation routines are sometimes referred to as "shrink" and "stretch" routines, respectively. With shrink and stretch routines, athletes feel ready to handle less than optimal circumstances.

Simulations: Expecting the unexpected

A key characteristic that distinguishes between more and less effective athletes is being able to maintain one's focus in the face of adversity. Athletes learn to do this in several ways. First, they develop their mental and emotional management skills. However, they do not stop there. Athletes then practice these skills in situations that are increasingly stressful and/or distracting. Simulation training is often used to accomplish this and involves having athletes and teams practice in environments that are as similar to the competitive environment as possible—similar physically (e.g., practice in humid environment if will be playing in one), mentally (e.g., practice with loud crowd noise played on loudspeaker system if playing in a noisy arena), and emotionally (e.g., with someone judging and scoring practices). Hence, coaches have shot putters practice while distracting camera clicks are going off, have figure skaters do run-throughs in their performance attire with an audience present, and conduct basketball training sessions that end with scrimmages where a referee is on the court with the clock running and an actual score is on the scoreboard. Practicing in simulated stressful situations like these help athletes and teams become used to the pressure and also learn to expect the unexpected. That is, they can anticipate what might occur in atypical situations and develop effective preparation and coping responses. In addition, there is evidence that practicing under stressful conditions (where the level of stress is challenging, but not overwhelming) facilitates athletes' mental preparation and coping strategies. Such practice also reduces uncertainty, a major source of stress in competitive sport.

Although real-life simulation is ideal, imagined experience (i.e., using mental imagery) can also help athletes to prepare for adversity. For example, one Olympic champion indicated that early in her career, people told her not to become nervous at the Olympic Games—just think of the Olympic competition as another practice. She found that for her that was impossible to do. So instead, in practice she would imagine what it felt like to be nervous at the Olympics, vividly recalling the racing of her heart, dry mouth, and nervous thoughts. Then, she would practice getting used to and controlling these anxiety-driven emotions, effectively developing coping strategies.

Imagery can be a powerful technique for simulating a wide range of circumstances in practice (e.g., imagine running neck and neck with an opponent in the last 50 m of the 400 m dash, defending power plays in hockey, holding an unexpected lead on an opponent in a close contest) and provides a great training ground for mental preparation. It is important to remember, however, that when using imagery to simulate situations that all the senses (e.g., visual, auditory, kinesthetic) should be used, that it needs to be consistently employed, and that an internal (seeing it from the performer's) and external (seeing it from a spectator's) perspective should be considered.

Team mental preparation

Coaches frequently talk about mentally preparing their teams. It is quite surprising, then, that this area has seldom been studied by sport psychology researchers. The previously mentioned team efficacy research certainly informs efforts in this area, as does research on whether group cohesion influences sport performance. In particular, the research shows that the more cohesive a team, the better the team's performance, the lower its anxiety, and the higher its confidence. Team cohesion, then, is an important mental preparation consideration. Related to cohesion are team-building efforts where sport psychologists work with teams to increase their levels of trust and communication. They also try to enhance cohesion by identifying common goals, clarifying roles, and facilitating social support.

These research findings imply that in developing team mental preparation procedures, team efficacy and cohesion must be considered. For example, some individuals on a team may prefer to be very social, and laugh and joke around as part of their mental preparation, whereas others like to sit quietly by themselves. Team cohesion could be negatively affected if athletes do not understand these intrateam differences (e.g., not everyone psychs up the same way) and coaches may find it useful to group athletes by their social–emotional preferences in pregame locker rooms so those who want to be social do not interfere with those who would like to have things quiet. Individual athletes should also realize that they should adapt their routine, at times, to fit in with general team preparation (e.g., participating in a team meeting before the game rather than being alone). Finally, teams may need to engage in rituals (e.g., team huddle and chant before the game) that help enhance overall efficacy and cohesion in their pregame mental preparation.

It is more than mental preparation

Mental preparation is not the only critical factor that determines performance success. Research in high performance sporting environments reveals that a number of social, organizational, and political stresses are placed on individual athletes and teams. Hence, in addition to optimal mental preparation, they need to develop a variety of coping and self-regulation skills to deal with these many stressors. For this reason, it is critical to remember that mental preparation is absolutely necessary, but alone, not sufficient for peak performance and learning. Mental preparation must always be viewed within the larger social and motivational climates where athletes and teams exist.

Summary

Mental preparation is critical to sport success and involves efforts to mentally prepare for both competitions and practices. Sport psychology research has identified a number of mental preparation principles that can be used to guide practice in this important area. These principles include recognizing the importance of mental preparation for competitions and practices, identifying one's zone of optimal functioning, developing emotional management skills, ensuring that mental preparation routines enhance confidence, realizing the importance of focusing on process and performance goals in mental preparation, developing and adhering to competition and practice routines, using simulation training to test and further revise mental preparation routines, and remembering that team mental preparation is just as important as individual mental preparation. The key, however, is to integrate these principles into mental preparation routines and procedures—into practical and simple strategies that athletes and coaches can employ systematically. The case studies that follow show how these general principles can be used systematically and customized to meet individual needs and the specific performance context.

CASE STUDIES

Although principles and best practices involving mental preparation for individual athletes and teams can and should be identified, helping athletes and teams optimally prepare is a complex process influenced by a variety of factors. The best way to help athletes or teams mentally prepare is influenced by the particular setting in which they perform, their performance history, and their personality. Hence, an effective way to better understand how to help athletes optimally mentally prepare is to examine individual case studies. Four case studies follow and demonstrate how sport psychology consultants can help athletes and teams with mental preparation.

CASE STUDY 1: PRACTICING WITH PURPOSE

Athlete/coach/team
Coach G. was a highly experienced junior national baseball coach. He had a talented but young team.

Background/reason for consultancy
Although his players were highly motivated when it came to games, Coach G. was concerned because they did not approach on-the-field, batting cage, and strength and conditioning practices with the same intensity.

Professional assessment
Based on his extensive experience, it was also clear to Coach G. that despite his team's talent, they could not win the conference championship without having big improvements in their practice intensity. As part of the team's normal mental training program, then, Coach G. asked a sport psychology consultant to focus special attention on helping his players practice with purpose and intensity.

Intervention
The consultant had worked with this team before, but practice intensity had not been a focus. So as part of the first mental

CASE STUDIES (Continued)

training session for the season, the consultant held a group discussion and had the players identify what things great teams do, or characteristics they possess, that allow them to become great. Characteristics that were generated included such things as having confidence and trust in one another, making good decisions, having good team cohesion, and engaging in peer coaching. With probing and by questioning certain players, the consultant made sure practicing with purpose, norms of productivity, and initiative were identified. These were defined and discussed with the athletes. Finally, each team member graded himself and the team on a 1 (not at all) to 10 (very much so) rating scale for each item. The team indicated that practice intensity was a six, falling somewhere between the highest-rated item (confidence) and lowest-rated item (engaging in peer coaching).

This activity suggested a disparity between the coaches' and the players' perceptions of their level of practice intensity and purpose, so a session was scheduled to discuss the importance of the topic. The coach shared his views on the importance of practice intensity and the consultant gave examples of high-status athletes who were known for their practice focus and intensity (e.g., Tiger Woods, Michael Jordan). The best player on the team's high level of practice intensity was pointed out and discussed. This was important because focusing on practice intensity does little good if only the coaching staff thinks it is important—the team must perceive it as a significant issue.

The team was then asked how they could practice with more purpose and intensity. What emerged were strategies that could be focused on—some identified by the team and others by the coach and consultant. The strategies that were derived included:

1. Setting specific daily goals for practice.
2. Taking a few minutes before practice to settle oneself and mentally prepare for the session.
3. Developing several refocusing strategies that could be used if any of the athletes became distracted in practice.
4. Giving permission to each other to discuss what should be said if one teammate sees that another is not focusing and working hard.
5. Providing weekly feedback as to the level of practice purpose and intensity exhibited by the team.

Outcome

These strategies were perceived as successful by Coach G. relative to increasing his team's practice intensity and sense of purpose. Practice intensity was much better than it had been before the program. However, it never made it to the level Coach G. had hoped and it was his conclusion that in addition to the mental preparation being provided, he needed to place more emphasis on recruiting key players who are not only highly skilled, but will bring a sense of purpose and practice intensity to the program.

CASE STUDY 2: THE CASE OF PREPERFORMANCE ROUTINES—HELPING JONNY PERFORM MORE CONSISTENTLY

Athlete

Jonny was a highly talented international male mogul freestyle skier. An intelligent male in his early 20s at the time of the consultation, Jonny was highly motivated to be successful and worked very hard, but was somewhat free spirited and cavalier in his approach.

Background

The sport psychology consultant encountered Jonny while working with the national freestyle ski team. Jonny agreed to work with the sport psychology consultant and did so for 18 months.

Reason for consultancy

Though Jonny was talented, he was very inconsistent. One week he would win a World Cup event and the next he would finish out of the top 10. His coaches felt Jonny was very "scattered" in his approach to mental preparation and suggested that he work with the team's mental training coach.

Professional assessment

After an initial meeting the consultant verified the nature of the problem. Jonny was frustrated with his performance inconsistency and wanted to become a more consistent competitor. However, he made little association between his free-wheeling approach and his inconsistent performances.

Intervention

Right from the start, Jonny committed to the mental training program and made a conscious effort to improve his mental preparation. He met regularly with the sport psychology consultant and also an assistant coach, who, with Jonny's permission, was in close contact with the consultant. The first strategy that was employed with Jonny was for him to become more organized and develop a preperformance routine. During his meetings with the consultant, Jonny was asked to identify, discuss, and contrast the differences in his mental and physical preparation for his most and least successful past performances. Based on patterns identified from this retrospective comparison, a preperformance routine was developed. This involved Jonny setting aside time to relax on the day of competition by watching his favorite DVD or going for a walk. He also would use centered breathing (taking a slow deep breath) to relax in the chair lift between runs and would repeat key phrases and words such as "chest up" or "perspective" to himself. Jonny also used his centered breathing anywhere from two to five times in the starting gate just before he would leave. Finally, once on top of the hill, he made sure he followed the same physical stretching and warm-up preparation routine before every race.

It is important to note that Jonny did not develop his final routine in 1 or 2 weeks. Rather, based on reflecting on his mental preparation used in previous good versus poor performances, a working routine was developed. He then used this routine and modified and added to it over time. Hence, by the time he reached the Olympics, Jonny had been working on developing a more consistent routine for over a year. Lastly, it is important to note that some of the routine components were developed from talking with the consultant, but other aspects were derived in collaboration with the assistant coach and/or through self-reflection by Jonny. The coaches also constantly reminded Jonny of the importance of being more consistent in his approach.

Outcome

Based on an informal analysis of his performances prior to and after his mental preparation work, and Jonny's and his coaches assessments of his efforts to improve his mental preparation, his sport psychology work paid off. He had a very successful career and won an Olympic medal.

Case study 3: Expecting the unexpected—developing shrink and stretch precompetitive routines

Athlete

Steve was a 28-year-old international wrestling competitor who had medaled at the World Championships and was expected to medal in the upcoming Olympic Games.

Reason for consultancy

The team's sport psychology consultant was approached by Steve because of his concern about his mental preparation. In the previous Olympics, he was unexpectedly beaten in the early round of the tournament.

Background

Steve indicated that in the previous Olympics, he had been optimally mentally prepared to compete while in the tunnel leading to the arena. He had done his usual normal 20 min physical warm-up doing the same exercises that he always did, engaging in shadow wrestling visualizing himself shooting takedowns and countering moves against his upcoming opponent, and engaging in light sparring with a teammate. He then had sat quietly for 5 min visualizing the match and reminding himself of wrestling his way—versus his opponent's way. However, as he was staying loose in the tunnel holding his optimal focus, the assistant coach had approached and indicated that the bout order had been changed to accommodate putting a home country athlete on prime time television. His match had been delayed. Steve remembers getting upset and saying: "This is the Olympics. How can they do this? This is bull _____!" Twenty minutes later, Steve was again in the tunnel awaiting his bout. However, he did not feel right and

wondered if they would delay the match again. He took the mat and performed poorly, unexpectedly losing to a less-skilled opponent. Steve indicated that his head had not been in the right place and it had cost him his Olympic Games.

Professional assessment

With Steve's permission, the consultant talked to his coach from the last Olympics and gained his perspective on the situation. Coach Johnson verified Steve's account of things. He agreed that the unexpected delay had disrupted Steve's mental preparation and focus, causing him to wrestle in an uncharacteristically lethargic manner, performing well below his potential.

Intervention

After talking to Steve, it was clear that he had a very definitive mental and physical preparation routine that he religiously followed before all matches. What he did not have were variants of his routine to deal with unexpected delays in competitive events (a stretch routine) or unexpected late arrival at the venue and corresponding minimization of the time needed to mentally prepare (a shrink routine).

The intervention began by having Steve write down exactly what he does to mentally prepare for each of his matches. Because wrestlers are likely to compete more than once per day, he began his preparation 1 h before his match. Steve and the consultant discussed his normal routine (Table 6.1.a) with the consultant providing a rationale for having consistent routines (e.g., research with Olympic athletes has consistently shown that more successful competitors have set routines and mentally prepare for all matches the same way). The discussion then turned to the fact that at times, unexpected things happen and matches either get delayed or athletes have less time than anticipated to prepare. A general discussion as to how one might deal with "shrink" and "stretch" mental preparation situations ensued. In the "shrink" situation, Steve outlined what he would mentally and physically do if he had only 10 min to get ready for a match (Table 6.1.b), whereas in the "stretch" situation, he outlined a strategy for holding his focus over time (Table 6.1.c).

Writing shrink and stretch mental preparation routines down on a sheet or paper and executing them in competition are two different things, however. So, working with Steve's coach, the consultant had him field test each routine in a practice match environment. He even tried his shrink routine (pretending he had only 10 min to get ready) in an international dual meet. This allowed him to make minor modifications to these emergency routines and gave him confidence that they would work.

Outcome

Steve performed well at the next Olympic Games, earning a silver medal. He experienced no unexpected changes in his preparatory time before matches. Hence, he did not need to

CASE STUDIES (Continued)

Table 6.1 Olympic wrestler's normal (a), shrink (b), and stretch (c) mental preparation routines.

(a) Normal routine	(b) Shrink routine	(c) Stretch routine
Get dressed 1 h before match	Review strategic goals while being transported to venue	Ask coach to monitor situation to keep apprised of when bout likely to begin
Review strategic goals for bout	Try to do some light arm stretches while being transported	Don't watch other matches if multiple mats are involved
Stretch and do some light running	As soon as arrive at venue, have the coach find out exactly how long there is before the match begins while getting dressed as quickly as possible	If it looks like a long delay, find quiet location near mat and distract self by listening to music
Engage in light sparring with teammate while visualizing shooting and countering moves on upcoming opponent		
Sit quietly while listening to music, purposefully ignoring other matches	Stretch and engage in light sparring with teammate while visualizing shooting and countering moves on upcoming opponent	Don't sit more than 10 min without getting up and some moving around
At approximately 15 min before the match, activate self with stretching and shadow wrestling		Once receive estimate of when the match will start activate self with stretching and shadow wrestling (or light sparring with teammate if time available)
Adjust singlet and take a deep centering breath before taking mat saying "win or take me off on a shield" before shaking hands with the opponent	Activate self, adjust singlet, and take a deep centering breath before taking mat saying "win or take me off on a shield" before shaking hands with the opponent	Activate self, adjust singlet, and take a deep centering breath before taking mat saying "win or take me off on a shield" before shaking hands with the opponent

use his shrink or stretch routines. However, in the Olympic Trials, one of the wrestlers performing before his semi-finals match sustained a serious neck injury and had to be taken off the mat on a stretcher, causing a 20-min delay in his start time. At first, this unexpected circumstance disrupted Steve's focus, but he then remembered his stretch routine and focused on implementing it. He was successful in doing so and beat his opponent. Equally important, Steve now had the confidence that he could deal with unexpected events and optimally prepare mentally regardless of the situation. This was a big relief to Steve going into the Olympic Games.

CASE STUDY 4: TEAM PREPARATION–ROUTINES AND SIMULATION

Team
This was an all-star women's volleyball team that was preparing to compete in various national tournaments.

Reason for consultancy
Given the highly competitive nature of these competitions, the team wanted to refine their preparation so they would perform at their best, be consistent, and be able to adapt to unforeseeable situations.

Professional assessment
It was explained to the team that their performance would be more consistent if the team's prematch routine was consistent. Furthermore, if the routine helped each player to find her individual zone of optimal functioning (IZOF) and be mentally prepared, the prematch routine would also improve performance

too. Because of the individual differences between players, and the brief time the team had to bond, the consultant thought that the team would play at its best if the routine were highly individualized. If every *player* were at her best, and dedicated to working together, then the *team* would be at its best. As such, the objective of the sport psychology intervention was to develop consistent, purposeful, and individualized precompetition routines that could be integrated into overall team preparation procedures.

Intervention
The team's routine was developed by assessing three pieces of information: (i) individual zones of optimal functioning (which represented the end-goal for each routine); (ii) the psychological coping skills and strategies of each player; and (iii) the physical and group needs of the team. These three pieces of information were integrated to create the team routine. The team/physical demands created a timeline that provided a framework or structure. Within that framework, individual mental skills and team activities were applied to help get each player into her "zone" and be mentally prepared.

Players reflected on (previous) good performances to complete a "mental toolbox" form, and to identify characteristics of their individual zones. The toolbox helped each player to create an inventory of effective skills that they already had—such as self-talk, mental imagery, effective goals, and ways to control energy (i.e., energizing and relaxing). Because most of the players did not have effective ways to relax and refocus during competitions, they developed centering techniques. The team also developed imagery scripts based on previous best-ever performances that helped each athlete to feel more confident, focused, and "in the

CASE STUDIES (Continued)

zone." These scripts, referred to as "personal highlight reels," varied from 10 s to 2 min in length. The highlight reels could be applied at various times of times before or during each match. The women had great self-talk skills, strategies to get pumped-up, and ways to use goals to help them perform better, so they did not invest time to develop those skills. However, the team was frequently reminded to use the skills that they had already developed.

The coaches developed a timeline in consultation with the players, the consultant, and the team's exercise physiologist. The team would arrive at the venue and "check in" 90 min before the match to make sure everyone was on time. The girls had 15 min to chat, relax, listen to music, etc. Seventy-five minutes before the match, everyone would get together to "fuel up" (nutrition), receive their uniforms, manage injuries (taping, etc.), discuss tactics (led by coach), and reflect on their individual goals for the match and the warm-up. This attention to detail helped everyone feel prepared and assured. The team's warm-up began 45 min before the match, and it included drills to increase core temperature, stretch muscles, rehearse volleyball skills, and work together. Players were advised to control the tempo of their warm-up, using it to relax or to get more pumped up, depending on their individual needs (like controlling their thermostats). Players could take short breaks from the 40-min warm-up to

visualize or do other mental preparation routines. Throughout the entire prematch routine, players were encouraged to be talkative. This helped everyone feel connected and energized, and it encouraged positive communication during the match. The last 3 min of the warm-up was "own time," where every player could do whatever she needed to get completely into her zone. Some players spent this time alone, some were in pairs, and others formed small groups (e.g., the "talkers"). Finally, after the warm-up (5-min before the start of the match), everyone came together for a team huddle. In the huddle, players were given a moment to clear their heads, the coach gave a confidence-building and informational (but simple) speech, a team "cheer" was done, and official formalities were executed.

Outcome

Focusing on their mental preparation helped this team perform more consistently. Ironically, the players felt that thinking more about their performance *before* each match helped them to think less during the match—they could "zone out and just do it." The coaches and athletes were so satisfied with how they performed that the following year, they extended their preparation to include 3-day-long precompetition routines, brief prepractice routines, and coping strategies specifically aimed to turn things around during a bad game or practice.

References

Gould, D., Guinan, D., Greenleaf, C., Medbery, R., Peterson, K. (1999) Factors affecting Olympic performance: perceptions of athletes and coaches from more and less successful teams. *The Sport Psychologist* **13**, 371–395.

Greenleaf, C., Gould, D., Dieffenbach, K. (2001) Factors influencing Olympic performance: interviews with Atlanta and Nagano U.S. Olympians. *Journal of Applied Sport Psychology* **13**, 154–184.

Further reading

Hanin, Y.L. (2000) *Emotions in Sport*. Human Kinetics, Champaign.

Jones, G., Hanton, S., Cinnaughton, D. (2007) A framework for mental toughness in the world's best performers. *The Sport Psychologist* **21**, 243–264.

Orlick, T. (1986) *Psyching for Sport: Mental Training for Athletes*. Human Kinetics, Champaign.

Weinberg, R.S., Gould, D. (2007) *Foundations of Sport and Exercise Psychology*. 4th Edn. Human Kinetics, Champaign.

Chapter 7
Enhancing team effectiveness

Albert V. Carron[1], Shauna M. Burke[2] and Kim M. Shapcott[3]

[1]School of Kinesiology, University of Western Ontario, London, Ontario, Canada
[2]Bachelor of Health Sciences Program, University of Western Ontario, London, Ontario, Canada
[3]School of Kinesiology, University of Western Ontario, London, Ontario, Canada

Introduction

A useful starting point in gaining an understanding of groups is the paradoxical suggestion that each group is like every other group, like some other groups, and like no other group. Certainly the initial and the final components of the statement are seemingly contradictory. However, both components are correct.

Consider the last component of the statement (i.e., each group is like no other group). Members of a family could argue that their family has few parallels with any of the other groups to which they belong. For example, family members might point out that compared to their sport teams, work groups, or social groups, their family is closer (or more dysfunctional), more (or less) efficient in achieving its objectives, and so on. In fact, members of that same family might even argue that their family doesn't even bear a resemblance to other families. They might point out, for example, that the nature of interactions and communications (including the quality and quantity) that occur in their family are unique.

That any group is like every other group is also easily illustrated. For example, every group, including a family, a sport team, and a work crew, develops a structure that is made up of four components. These four components contribute to the

Sport Psychology. 1st edition. Edited by Britton Brewer.
Published 2009 by Blackwell Publishing.
ISBN 978-1-4051-7363-6.

stability of the group and help to differentiate a true group from a collection of strangers. One of those components is a *status* hierarchy. Individuals in any group possess a wide variety of different attributes. Some—*ascribed attributes*—are characteristics the individual possesses that are not the result of personal effort; for example, ethnicity, religion, and gender. Other attributes—*achieved attributes*—on the contrary are attained through personal effort; for example, skill, education, and prior experience. In different groups, different types of achieved and ascribed attributes are valued differently—depending on the group and its purposes. Being the Chief Executive Officer (CEO) of a major corporation might bring considerable prestige to an individual in work and social groups. However, if that CEO finds himself/herself stuck in the wilderness because of a plane crash, he/she would find that the individual who has the best survival skills would have the most status. As individuals begin to interact in any group situation, those who possess valued attributes are identified and accorded more status.

Group *roles* are another structural component common to all groups. Members of all groups develop a generalized expectation for those individuals who through ability or experience assume specific responsibilities. A typical responsibility (role) that is characteristic of all groups is leader but other less formal roles (e.g., peacemaker, social catalyst, group comic) develop in most groups.

Group *norms* are the third component of group structure. A family, a sport team, a work group, a military unit, a social group, and so on, develop generalized expectations for the behavior of group members. These norms might be related to common expectations for work output, civility in the interactions and communications among members, or punctuality and attendance at group functions. All groups develop norms around matters considered important by their members.

Finally, in every group, members occupy specific *positions*. For example, generally, family members sit at the same place at dinner and occupy the same chair in the living room. In businesses, employees have specific locations for eating, working, and meeting. The knowledge and acceptance of positional stability by group members contribute to the development of the group.

In this chapter, we capitalize on the principle that every group is like all other groups in order to advance a number of generalizations that have evolved from published research. Space restrictions limit what we can discuss, so we have focused on some of the constructs that have the most application to Olympic teams, be they sport teams or medical groups. These are group size, group status, group cohesion, group roles, and group goals. In our discussion of these five group constructs, we introduce the research-based generalizations and then provide some suggestions for their application in groups.

Group size

The Olympic Games pose a unique challenge with regard to team selection and, in particular, team size. Most countries have their own governing bodies that develop and implement policies that regulate the selection process. These guidelines usually stipulate the maximum number of athletes that can be retained for each sport. However, there is some flexibility in the exact number of athletes on a given team or staff in support groups.

Decisions about group size do matter. Independent of the nature of the situation (e.g., sport teams, business groups, social groups), members of larger groups are less satisfied with their group experience than members of smaller groups. In addition, members experience a decrease in participation

and feelings of responsibility for the group's welfare. Furthermore, a larger group size results in less interaction and communication between athletes and coaches and/or staff and leaders. It also reduces opportunities for individuals to contribute significantly to the group's performance.

A larger group size does not have a negative impact solely on psychosocial factors. *Social loafing*—the reduction in individual effort witnessed when individuals work in groups compared to when they work alone—also represents a problem in larger groups. Intuitively, it seems improbable that social loafing would be a concern in the context of the Olympic Games. The strong commitment that Olympians make to their sport through countless years of training and sacrifices should keep motivation sufficiently high to ward off social loafing. However, research has found that Olympic athletes are not immune to social loafing. For instance, researchers observed that social loafing in Olympic rowers increased when group size increased (some specific suggestions for limiting social loafing are discussed later).

Increased group size is also associated with reduced group cohesion. One explanation for this finding is that as group size increases it becomes more difficult to communicate effectively and coordinate team activities.

Optimal group size

When it comes to group size, some coaches err on the side of caution and initially select too many athletes, whereas other coaches prefer to carry the minimum number of athletes. Several advantages and disadvantages have been identified by athletes for sport teams that are too small or too large. The main advantage of smaller teams is that athletes have more opportunities to compete; a disadvantage is lack of team depth. In contrast, an advantage of larger teams is an increase in depth. There are limits to the *size = depth* generalization; however, as group size continues to increase, the resources necessary for group effectiveness eventually plateau. Furthermore, large rosters make it difficult for coaches to communicate effectively with athletes, so athlete–coach interactions suffer. Consequently, an increase in group size translates to a decrease in effective coordination of resources. These findings highlight the need for coaches to determine the ideal team size for optimal performance in their sport.

Three explicit suggestions have been advanced by researchers about the optimal group size for work groups, such as medical support teams at the Olympic Games. The first is that *five members* represent the optimal size. With an odd number, a deadlock is not possible, a split does not produce a social isolate (i.e., as would be the case with a group of three), generally sufficient resources are available to carry out the group task, and members can shift roles easily and withdraw from awkward positions without undue hardship.

The second suggestion is that group organizers should strive to determine a *functional or critical group size*. This involves more art than science. An organizing committee must determine the point at which the group possesses adequate resources to carry out its task. As the number of group members increases beyond this functional/critical complement, the number of individuals not actively participating also increases.

The third suggestion relates directly to sport teams. To satisfy the principle of *functional or critical group size*, a sufficient number of individuals should be retained in order to practice efficiently and effectively. When possible, it is beneficial that resources are available to scrimmage in team sports and compete in individual sports. This allows for opportunities for personal instruction, reinforcement, and individual participation, and contributes to stronger feelings of commitment and accountability to the group.

Practical suggestions

Optimal group size varies from sport to sport and from team to team. For example, 10 athletes are needed for a scrimmage in basketball, 12 in volleyball, and 22 in football (soccer). In addition, specific policies pertaining to team selection for the Olympic Games can hinder a coaching staff's ability to completely control team size. Having said this, all coaches and organizers have to bear in mind that smaller is better than larger. When a larger roster is inevitable, various team building strategies (which will be discussed later) should be used to enhance cohesion in order to counterbalance the negative effects of group size.

As was discussed earlier, social loafing has a tendency to increase with increases in group size. Strategies that can be used to reduce social loafing include: (a) monitor and independently evaluate individual behavior in group situations; (b) outline the importance or meaningfulness of each team members contribution; and (c) insure that each group member is highly familiar with all other group members.

These conditions provide insight into potential strategies to combat the problem. Specifically, social loafing increases when an individual's output cannot be evaluated independently, the task is not perceived to be very meaningful, the individual does not identify with the task or group outcomes, other individuals in the situation are strangers, and the individual perceives his/her contributions as redundant.

Group status

When different individuals come together and begin to interact, a number of similarities become evident, as do a wide range of differences. In any group, status differences are inevitable—they emerge because individuals hold different beliefs, perceptions, and/or evaluations about the importance of various attributes or personal characteristics. In turn, these beliefs, perceptions, and/or evaluations influence the dynamics (i.e., the expectations and interactions) among group members.

Importance of status congruency

The presence of differences in status in any group does not necessarily imply that group effectiveness will suffer. Instead, a lack of *consensus* or *agreement* regarding the status rankings or placement within a group has the potential to be particularly detrimental to overall team effectiveness. Typically, a lack of consensus arises from a discrepancy in a group member's perceptions about where he/she is *currently* in the status hierarchy relative to personal perceptions about where he/she *belongs*.

On an Olympic team, status hierarchies can be either formal (i.e., differences in status associated with being a team captain versus a co-captain or an assistant captain versus a team member) or informal (i.e., differences in status associated with having relatively more or less ability). Team effectiveness is influenced by two types of *status congruency*. One pertains to the degree of congruence between the formal and informal status hierarchies. A team will be more effective if athletes with a high formal status (e.g., team captains) are the same athletes who possess a high level of informal status within the group. The second pertains to the degree of congruence between where an athlete sees him/herself in the status hierarchy and where the team sees the athlete. A team will be more effective if athletes have an accurate perception of their place in the status hierarchy—and possibly most importantly, the importance of a status hierarchy is downplayed.

Practical suggestions

Insofar as the congruence between formal and informal status hierarchies is concerned, four scenarios are possible: (i) the same individuals possess the highest formal and informal status and the source of that status is positive (e.g., the best athlete is the team captain and he/she possesses an exceptional work ethic); (ii) the same individuals possess the highest formal and informal status but the source of that status is negative (i.e., the best athlete is the team captain, but he/she is a "party animal"); (iii) different individuals have the highest formal and informal status and the source of their status is positive (e.g., the best athlete and the team captain are not the same individual; both possess positive personal attributes); and (iv) different individuals have the highest formal and informal status but the source of status for at least one of them is negative (e.g., the best athlete is not the team captain; one or both of them possesses a poor work ethic).

Obviously Option (i) is highly desirable and if this situation is present, the status quo ought to be preserved. If Option (ii) exists, a few strategies are possible. One is to remove the formal leadership role from the individual and the other is to remove the individual from the team. The latter may seem like an ivory tower suggestion because

when countries (and their teams) are striving for an Olympic medal or another challenging goal, it seems counterintuitive to cut a top athlete. Nonetheless, a cancer should not be permitted to grow until it poisons the whole organism.

In the case of Option (iii), it is recommended that the coaching staff include the high informal status athlete into a leadership role, and/or include him/her in the leadership process. Finally, in the case of Option (iv), the best course of action is to remove the individual from the team, regardless of the fact that he/she may possess a great deal of talent and ability. As indicated earlier, such an action may seem excessive but the negative behavior(s) of the athlete combined with the influential position of high informal status could have a negative impact on the behavior and attitudes of other team members, resulting in decreased team effectiveness.

As was pointed out earlier, it is also possible that there may not be congruence between where an athlete sees him/herself in the status hierarchy and where the team or coach sees that individual. Who takes the last shot in a close basketball game? It is possible for some athletes to feel insulted if their coach chooses a teammate.

A useful strategy implemented by many top coaches is to discuss a number of potential team-disrupting situations in an open forum comprised of all team members. Questions are used as a catalyst for discussion: "How should you or your teammates respond if I make a substitution you don't like?" "How can we preserve team unity if you're not one of the athletes chosen for the dress roster or the starting lineup?" Athletes who make a commitment in a situation far removed from the excitement of competition have a greater tendency to honor that commitment in competitive situations.

Group cohesion

Cohesion is defined as a dynamic process which is reflected in the tendency for a group to stick together and remain united in the pursuit of its instrumental objectives and/or for the satisfaction of member affective needs. The term "cohesion"—often used interchangeably with "team unity" and "team chemistry"—is the most important group variable. In fact, recent research has revealed that team cohesion is considered, by both Olympic athletes and coaches, to be a major factor influencing team success. Olympic athletes participating in both team and individual sports deem cohesion and team building strategies to be essential to success. Furthermore, team unity is perceived to be one of the few factors that differentiate successful from unsuccessful Olympic teams. In fact, historically, lack of cohesion has been cited as the main reason why talented teams have failed to bring home the Olympic gold. For example, after the disastrous performances by the so-called Dream Teams—the 2004 US Olympic Men's basketball team and the 2006 Canadian Olympic Men's hockey team—it was suggested that the failure to develop the necessary team chemistry accounted for the lack of medal success.

Cohesion is *multidimensional* in nature in that there are numerous factors that cause a group to remain united, and these factors can differ from group to group. In sport teams, the two strongest factors are the task and social relationships. Task cohesion refers to being united in achieving the team's objectives, whereas social cohesion refers to the quality of social relationships present. Both task cohesion and social cohesion contribute to team performance (although the former is slightly more important).

Correlates of cohesion

Cohesion has been found to be correlated with environmental factors, personal factors, leadership factors, and team factors. It is important to note that the relationships between cohesion and these correlates may be (are likely) reciprocal. For example, cohesion is correlated with collective efficacy (i.e., a shared belief regarding the group's ability to succeed at a given task). It is probable that cohesion increases collective efficacy and collective efficacy increases cohesiveness. A brief overview of some of the research findings from within each of the four categories is discussed in the following section.

Environmental factors

Several environmental factors—group size, level of competition, and geographical considerations—have been found to be related to cohesion. For

Olympic teams, physical and functional proximity is of particular interest. Olympic teams are often faced with the decision of whether to centralize (i.e., to come together in a single location) for training prior to the Olympic Games. Research has found that when individuals within a group are brought into close proximity, there is more opportunity to interact and communicate about task and social issues which results in an increase in cohesiveness. The 2006 Canadian Olympic Women's hockey team provides an excellent example of the benefits of proximity with regard to cohesion. Leading up to the Olympics, the Canadian team centralized for over half a year—practicing, training, competing, and living together. In comparison, the American team only held periodic camps before road trips and exhibition games. The Canadian team won the gold medal and players attributed their success to a high level of cohesion resulting from centralization.

Personal factors

There is also a link between cohesion and an individual athlete's cognitions, affect, and behavior. Specifically, cohesion is correlated with state anxiety, individual satisfaction, individual effort, sacrifice behavior, and adherence behavior. The link between cohesion and state anxiety is of particular interest for Olympians. The Olympics involve performing on a world stage under the watchful eyes of millions. This can be an anxiety-inducing event for most athletes, and cohesion can counteract this anxiety. Athletes who perceive their team to be high in task and social cohesion report lower levels of both somatic and cognitive anxiety. Furthermore, athletes higher in task cohesion perceive their cognitive and state anxiety symptoms as more facilitative ("I am anxious, but that is a sign that I am ready").

Leadership factors

Two elements of leadership that are related to the development of group cohesion are the leader's decision style and the leader's behavior. Research has consistently found that cohesion is more likely to develop when a more democratic coaching style is employed (i.e., the coach encourages athlete participation in decisions related to the team). Concerning coaching behaviors, teams exhibit higher levels of task and social cohesion when coaches engage in training and instruction, social support, and positive feedback. In fact, Olympians have mentioned coaching as a major factor affecting performance. Specifically, coach contact, trust, feedback, and focus on creating a team climate have all been cited as critical to successful performance.

Team factors

Numerous team factors have been linked to cohesion. In particular, cohesion has been found to be correlated with various aspects of roles, norms, collective efficacy, and performance. Team success is the factor most commonly associated with cohesion. Research as found that both task and social cohesion are positively related to team success, and that team success is positively related to both task and social cohesion. Thus, highly successful teams are more likely to develop a sense of togetherness. On the contrary, unsuccessful teams that begin to develop greater cohesiveness should increase their chances of becoming successful.

Practical suggestions: Team building strategies

As mentioned earlier, creating a cohesive team is not an easy task. This is especially true for teams that are assembled only months prior to the Games or other important competitions. Fortunately, there are numerous team building strategies that can be implemented to increase the cohesiveness of a team in a relatively short amount of time. These strategies involve, for example, producing a positive team environment, working toward conformity to team norms, insuring role clarity and acceptance, and establishing team goals.

Team environment

Cohesion is enhanced by fostering feelings of distinctiveness and togetherness. Providing the team with unique identifiers (e.g., warm-up suits) or emphasizing unique traditions and/or history

associated with the team's country or location of origin highlights the presence of team distinctiveness and contributes to team unity. As mentioned earlier, cohesion can also be enhanced by togetherness which can be established by repeatedly placing team members in close physical proximity, such as centralization prior to the Olympic Games.

Team norms

Striving for conformity to important team norms is another method used to enhance team cohesion. A three-step intervention can be used to increase the likelihood that team members accept, internalize, and comply with team norms. First, a sense of ownership for the norms must be created. Second, athletes must recognize that the norms exist and see others following them. Third, team members must understand how the norms help accomplish the group's goals.

In some international teams (e.g., British Lions rugby team), the intervention is achieved in a day-long, pre-competition session. In small discussion groups, athletes identify important elements/behaviors that should be included in a team code of conduct. Through discussion, consensus is reached on the most important components; these are then brought forward and presented to the total group. Again, through discussion, consensus is reached in the total group on the most important components. The process—encouraging individual contributions, group discussions, and group consensus—helps to insure that individual athletes are committed to (and pressured into) honoring the agreed-upon code.

The role dimension

In its most common usage, a role is a part or character in a play or movie. In sociological, psychological, industrial, and sport contexts, it refers to a pattern of behavior expected of an individual. The two viewpoints are similar, of course. Audiences, such as members of any group, have general expectations for the pattern of behavior of actors playing a role (e.g., King Lear). If the actor's interpretation differs dramatically from those expectations, the audience response is characterized by dissatisfaction.

Types of roles

Roles are often categorized according to whether they relate to task (e.g., organizer) or social concerns (e.g., social catalyst), as well as to whether they are formal or informal in nature. A formal role is one prescribed by the group or organization (i.e., Coach, Director) whereas an informal role arises spontaneously as a result of interactions and communications within the group (i.e., team peacemaker). For example, in sport teams, these broad categorizations have been further subdivided into a myriad of specific responsibilities that athletes assume, for example, positional roles, formal and informal team leadership roles, social roles, communication roles, motivational roles, and organizational roles. Each individual athlete can have a variety of responsibilities, some of which they share with others. Moreover, over the life of a group, member responsibilities can change. Consequently, for any team to be effective, members must have a clear understanding of their role or roles. Unfortunately, this is not always the case.

A useful framework for understanding the dynamic nature of roles in teams is presented in Figure 7.1. In a team, the *role sender* (usually a coach) is responsible for communicating role responsibilities to the *focal person* (i.e., an athlete, another member of the coaching staff). For purposes of the present discussion, the process can be assumed to start with Event 1 when the role sender (the coach) develops specific expectations for the focal person (the athlete). Once those expectations are established, the role sender exerts pressure (Event 2) on the focal person to carry out the desired responsibilities. Event 3 then occurs; the focal person experiences the role expectation pressure and subsequently responds (Event 4).

The focal person's response, which can take many forms, is influenced by the situation. For example, a returning veteran athlete might immediately begin to carry out his/her role (role performance). Conversely, a young inexperienced athlete may experience confusion (role ambiguity), or be unwilling to accept the responsibilities prescribed (lack of role acceptance), or feel dissatisfaction or satisfaction (role dis/satisfaction), and so on.

It is possible that any of the three major principals included in Figure 7.1—the role sender, the

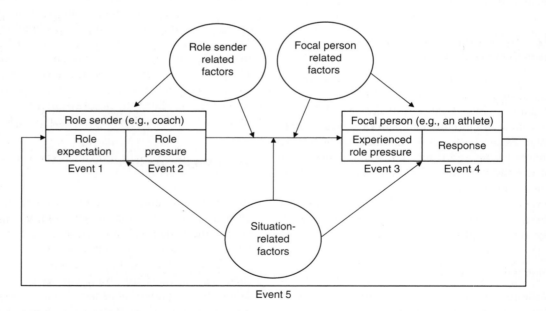

Figure 7.1. A theoretical framework of factors influencing the transmission and reception of role responsibilities.
Note: Adapted from Kahn, R.L., Wolfe, D.M., Quinn, R.P., Snoek, J.D., Rosenthal, R.A. (1964) *Organizational Stress: Studies in Role Conflict and Ambiguity*, p. 30. Wiley, New York

focal person, or the situation—could be a major problem in the communication of role responsibilities. An inexperienced coach may not be a good communicator. A non-starter athlete might not be a motivated listener. Time constraints (a situational factor) may reduce opportunities for communicating.

Athletes asked to identify reasons why they might not fully understand their role have offered a wide cross section of reasons. Some coaches do not communicate sufficiently, are not clear, and/or provide conflicting information. Also, some athletes do not have the capacity to understand instructions and/or fail to pay attention in practice. Finally, events such as changing positions and/or moving to a more elite level can produce confusion.

The role dimension is so important for effective group functioning that researchers have spent a considerable amount of time for studying correlates. For example, it has been shown that role ambiguity (a lack of understanding about role responsibilities) is associated with lower task cohesion, lower self-efficacy, reduced satisfaction, increased competitive anxiety, and an increased likelihood that the athlete will discontinue membership in the group. It has also been demonstrated that athletes who are more senior have greater role clarity than inexperienced athletes. However, these differences in role clarity can disappear over the course of a season.

Practical suggestions

Mike Keenan, a National Hockey League coach, has stated that in his attempts to foster a team-oriented philosophy, he has used frequent one-on-one meetings both on the ice and in the coach's room. Prior to meetings in the coach's room, it is useful to have both the coach and the athlete develop a list of the athlete's responsibilities. At the meeting, the player and coach compare perceptions, and any misconceptions by the athlete can be rectified. This approach may be time-consuming. If so, the coach can simply use the athlete's list of perceived responsibilities and either add or delete functions as appropriate.

Another approach used with some success is anonymous feedback to athletes from their teammates. Each team member is given a form containing the names of all his/her teammates. At the top of the sheet is the phrase "In order for us to be successful, XXXX must…" Each team member independently and confidentially writes statements about every other person on the team. After this process is completed, the statements are compiled and each team member receives a personal feedback summary that contains all the statements from the rest of the team.

A third approach that can be used to reduce role ambiguity is referred to as the *hot seat*. All team members are given an opportunity to publicly outline their responsibilities to their teammates. Each member is required to stand or sit in front of the group (i.e., the hot seat) and explain to the rest of the team what she/he believes his or her formal functions are. Following the presentation, teammates and coaches then agree with, modify, dispute, or add to the responsibilities listed by the athlete. The head coach has the final authority.

Group goals

Generally speaking, a goal represents a target, objective, standard, destination, or end toward which effort is directed. In addition, group (or team) goals represent *shared perceptions* regarding a desirable state of the group. The positive impact of goals on group achievement and success in both work and sport groups have been very well established. In fact, in many instances, group goals have been shown to be more strongly associated with team success than individual goals. In addition to reliable improvements in performance, group goals contribute to increased focus, direction, and motivation, as well as to greater perceptions of group cohesion, particularly if group member participation is encouraged.

Practical suggestions

When setting group goals, it has been suggested that the team—along with the coach and/or consultant—define the specific (target) areas in which goals are going to be set. A valuable means of identifying such areas is through the use of team performance profiling.

Team performance profiling

The overall aim of this exercise is to assess a team's primary strengths and weaknesses to facilitate group goal setting. The first step involves athletes working together to identify a complete list of the characteristics (physical, psychological, tactical) that are perceived to be most important for team success in their sport. The athletes then rate each of these characteristics on a scale of 1 (*not very important for team success*) to 10 (*most important for team success*), resulting in an "ideal score" for each characteristic. An alternative way to arrive at an "ideal score" is for athletes to collectively identify an "ideal" team (not their own), and to rank the characteristics that the athletes feel best describe this "ideal" team. In the second step of the exercise, athletes' rate their team's *current level* for each of the characteristics identified previously on a scale of 1 (*could not be any worse*) to 10 (*could not be any better*). This comprises a "current score" for each characteristic. The final step involves subtracting the current score for each characteristic from the ideal score, producing a "discrepancy score." The characteristic(s) identified as having the largest discrepancy values should then be targeted as areas for which group goals should be set. Engaging in the process of team performance profiling is advantageous, not only because it takes into consideration athletes' views on collective areas of concern, but also because specific target areas are identified, setting the stage for subsequent team goal setting.

Setting group goals

After approximately three or four specific target areas have been identified using the team profiling technique, the process of team goal setting can begin. Several principles are useful for coaches or sport leaders interested in establishing team goal setting programs. For example, group goals should be challenging, specific and quantitative (i.e., as opposed to vague, "do your best" goals), and realistic. Other principles for effective team goal setting include:

(a) Involving all members of the team in the goal setting process.

(b) Setting long-term goals first (e.g., for the training season) and short-term goals second (e.g., for each week). It may also be useful to utilize the small number of "target" areas identified using team performance profiling for setting short-term goals, and the remaining characteristics for the development of long-term goals.

(c) Developing specific strategies or "plans of action" that can be used to achieve the long-term goals (this will involve setting several short-term goals).

(d) Regularly monitoring progress and providing feedback related to team goals. It is helpful to display team goals and progress toward goals (e.g., team statistics) in a visible location such as a bulletin board outside of a locker room.

(e) Providing public praise for team progress. Sending out mass e-mails or newsletters highlighting team accomplishments are examples of possible avenues for openly praising progress toward and attainment of team goals.

(f) Fostering a sense of team confidence/ collective efficacy toward team goals. One means of enhancing collective efficacy is through the development of realistic expectations for team outcomes.

CASE STUDY

Group

Chris Smith, a young (33 years of age), highly successful college basketball coach has just been selected as Head Coach for the Utopia National Basketball Team for the upcoming Olympic Games. The Games will be held every 2 years. Chris's first contact with the team will be at a selection camp for 2 months.

Reason for consultancy

International experts believe that Chris has a difficult assignment. Despite high expectations at the previous Olympic Games, Utopia did poorly, finishing well out of the medals. One catalyst for the poor performance was an early upset. Another was the apparent presence of two cliques that formed around age and race differences. By the time the Olympics were over, members in the two opposing cliques were barely speaking to each other off the court. In debriefing sessions with the team members following the Olympic Games, three common themes surfaced: (i) communication among athletes and between athletes and the coaching staff, although never been very good at any time, disintegrated over the course of the Olympics; (ii) team task and social unity were virtually non-existent; and (iii) individual performance was often selfish and inconsistent with role responsibilities.

Background

Utopia is a country with relatively good basketball talent so 20 athletes have been invited to attend the selection camp. Among these twenty, eight are returnees from the team that competed in the previous Olympic Games. Four of the eight returnees are over 30 years of age and have represented Utopia at two previous Olympiads and one World Championship. All four are very close personally. One of the four was the captain of the previous Olympic team.

The Utopian Basketball Federation has suggested that Chris chose 15 athletes from the Selection Camp. These athletes will then continue to compete for positions on the team until 6 months prior to the Olympic Games. At that point, the final roster of 12 will be selected.

Questions for discussion

1. What steps could Chris take prior to the start of the Selection Camp to increase the chances for its success? Among possible courses of action, Chris could:

(a) Initiate personal contact with each of the 20 athletes before Selection Camp begins. Outline in general terms the reasons why the team was not successful in previous international competitions. Ask each athlete what could be done to overcome the problem(s). Have each athlete provided one specific step (behavior) that he/she will take to increase team cohesion.

(b) Specifically, plan social situations (i.e., room assignments, meals, and so on) so diversity in age, experience, and race are optimized. Convey both the plans and the reasons for these plans to the athletes.

2. What steps can Chris take at the start of the Selection Camp to increase the chances for its success? Among possible courses of action, Chris could:

(a) Begin camp with a day devoted to team building activities. Initially, have each athlete pair off with an unfamiliar other. Each athlete interviews the other and then in rotation introduces his/her partner to the total team.

(b) Have each pair of athletes establish a list of behaviors for on-court and off-court situations that will represent a "code of conduct" for the team. When each pair has completed the task, have them present the list to the total

group. Then have the total group determine the most critical behaviors that will constitute the code of conduct for the team.

3. What steps can Chris take during the Selection Camp to increase the chances for its success? Among possible courses of action, Chris could:

(a) As soon as possible, schedule one-on-one sessions and outline in detail the athlete's role (on and off the court) and the behaviors associated with that role. Obtain the athlete's commitment to that role and outline the consequences of a failure to carry out role expectations.

(b) Organize a team performance profiling/group goal setting session with all the athletes, encouraging active participation from the athletes in the goal setting process.

4. How can Chris insure that the cliques that were so destructive in the previous Olympiads do not reappear during the Selection Camp? Among possible courses of action, Chris could:

(a) Aim to effectively utilize the knowledge and experience of the eight returnees. Conduct a team meeting in which veteran players are encouraged to share what they learned from their previous Olympic experience with the new coaching staff and athletes. Ask all players for suggestions regarding how the mistakes that were made in the past can be avoided in the future.

5. A team can be defined as *a collection of individuals who possess a common identity, have common goals and objectives, share a common fate, develop structured patterns of interaction and communication, hold common perceptions about group norms, individual roles, individual status, and individual positions, possess a mutual respect and affection for one another, and consider themselves to be a team*. What preliminary steps can Chris take to insure that each of these components of the definition begins to appear during the Selection Camp? Among possible courses of action, Chris could:

(a) Have mandatory practice and training uniforms to encourage team distinctiveness outside of a game situation.

(b) Schedule regular team gatherings to ensure structured, consistent, and open communication among team members and coaching staff.

More background information

As a result of their performance at the Selection Camp, Chris selected the 15 athletes who will constitute The Utopia National Basketball Team for the 2 years leading up to the Olympics. Among the athletes selected are six returnees three of whom were starters. The returning players vary in age from 28 to 33 years, whereas all of the new players are under 23 years of age (including two 19-year-olds). Four of the returnees and six of the new players are members of one ethnic group; two returnees and three new players are members of another ethnic group.

CASE STUDY (Continued)

More questions for discussion

1. What further steps can Chris take to facilitate the development of task cohesion? Among possible courses of action, Chris could:

(a) Provide summary statistics from previous competition on important team outcome indices (e.g., turnovers, steals, and so on). In a group meeting, establish consensus

and agreement with regard to team goals for upcoming competitions.

2. What further steps can Chris take to facilitate the development of social cohesion? Among possible courses of action, Chris could:

(a) Periodically schedule specific team social functions (e.g., paint ball, team dinners, movies, and so on).

Further reading

Bull, S.J., Albinson, J.G., Shambrook, C.J. (1996) *The Mental Game Plan: Getting Psyched for Sport*. Sports Dynamics, Eastbourne.

Carron, A.V., Hausenblas, H.A., Eys, M.A. (2005) *Group Dynamics in Sport*, 3rd Edn. Fitness Information Technology, Morgantown.

Hackfort, D., Lidor, R., Duda, J. (2006) *Handbook of Research in Applied Sport Psychology*. Fitness Information Technology, Morgantown.

Hale, B., Collins, D. (2002) *Rugby Tough*. Human Kinetics, Champaign.

Janssen, J. (1999) *Championship Team Building: What Every Coach Needs to Know to Build a Motivated, Committed, and Cohesive Team*. Winning the Mental Game, Tucson.

Chapter 8
Injury prevention and rehabilitation

Britton W. Brewer

Department of Psychology, Springfield College, Springfield, MA, USA

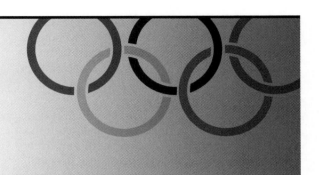

Introduction

Over the course of their sport careers, athletes spend thousands of hours training to strengthen their bodies, enhance their fitness, and prepare themselves physically for competition. Despite (and, in some cases, because of) this training, competitive athletes are at high risk for sustaining a sport injury. Across levels of sport involvement, sport injury is a common reason for hospital emergency room visits and constitutes a substantial public health concern in industrialized nations. Among elite performers, the injury rate in some sports eclipses 50% over a 1-year period. Sport injuries vary widely in both magnitude and duration of impact. Some injuries are minor and have little or no impact on sport training and competition, whereas other injuries are major and have a more pronounced effect on regular sport participation. Similarly, some injuries affect the ability of athletes to play their sports for only a short period of time, whereas other injuries keep athletes from participating in sport for a longer amount of time, possibly even permanently.

In addition to the obvious physical toll exacted by sport injuries, there are financial and psychological costs incurred by athletes who sustain injuries. Treatment costs, which can be particularly substantial when surgical procedures and extensive rehabilitation are involved, must be covered by the sport organization (e.g., team, national

Sport Psychology. 1st edition. Edited by Britton Brewer.
Published 2009 by Blackwell Publishing.
ISBN 978-1-4051-7363-6.

governing body [NGB]) or by the athletes themselves and their insurance or other mechanism. The financial impact of sport injuries can be magnified when athletes are unable to receive monetary compensation due to their inability to play their sport. From a psychological standpoint, sport injuries can hamper the ability of athletes to engage in behaviors central to success in their sport and, as a consequence, can produce responses in some athletes ranging from mild mood disturbance to clinically meaningful emotional distress.

Efforts directed at the prevention and treatment of sport injuries customarily have a decidedly physical emphasis. For example, strength and conditioning programs are sometimes implemented at least partially for the purpose of injury prevention, and physiotherapy is commonly prescribed to treat sport injuries. Based on a growing body of research linking psychological factors to both the occurrence of and recovery from sport injuries, however, psychological interventions have been developed and implemented for preventive and therapeutic purposes. Thus, methods of a psychological nature can be added to those used more traditionally in sports medicine to offer comprehensive services to athletes.

Injury prevention

Psychological antecedents of sport injury

In addition to anatomical, environmental, and other physical factors, psychological factors have been widely documented as contributing to the risk of sport injury occurrence. In particular, psychological stress has shown a robust association with the occurrence of injury across a variety of sports. In a series of more than 30 research investigations dating back to 1970, athletes reporting higher levels of stressful life events have consistently displayed a tendency to sustain more or more severe injuries. Common stressors include both positively and negatively perceived events in the personal, social, academic, occupational, and athletic lives of athletes.

In addition to life stress, other psychological factors that contribute to either the occurrence of sport injuries or sport participation time lost due to injury include various personality factors and coping resources. Among the personality characteristics that have been tied to sport injury outcomes are competitive trait anxiety, negative states of mind (e.g., anger, mood disturbance), and Type-A (e.g., aggressive, impatient, hard-driving) behavior, with athletes exhibiting higher levels of those characteristics experiencing elevated risk for more or more severe injuries. Social support is the coping resource that has been tied most frequently to sport injury. Low levels of perceived support from other people are associated with heightened vulnerability to sport injury.

Personality and coping resources affect sport injury risk not only directly but also by moderating the influence of life stress on sport injury outcomes. This means that they alter the magnitude of the relationship between life stress and the occurrence or severity of sport injuries. For example, the association between life stress and sport injury tends to be stronger for athletes high in competitive trait anxiety or low in social support than it is for athletes low in competitive trait anxiety or high in social support. Thus, the deleterious effects of life stress on sport injury occurrence or severity are exacerbated for athletes who are anxious about sport competition. Conversely, social support seems to have a buffering effect on the relationship between life stress and sport injury outcomes, as athletes high in social support are better able to experience high levels of life stress without incurring injury than are athletes low in social support.

The model depicted in Figure 8.1 represents an attempt to explain how psychological factors such as stressful events, personality, and coping resources can influence risk for incurring sport injury. Potentially stressful situations are thought to affect one's injury vulnerability through a process in which interpretations of the situations (i.e., cognitive appraisals) influence and are influenced by

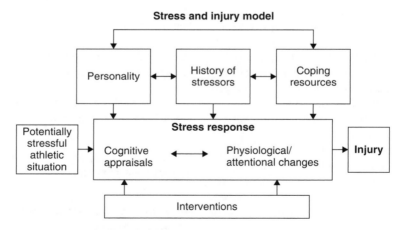

Figure 8.1. A model of stress and sport injury. *Source*: Williams, J.M. & Andersen, M.B. (1998) Psychosocial antecedents of sport injury: review and critique of the stress and injury model. *Journal of Applied Sport Psychology* **10**, 5–25. Reprinted with permission

physiological and attentional changes. The extent to which this stress response affects injury risk is itself influenced by any interventions directed at altering the stress response and the individual's personality, recent history of stressful life events, and coping resources. Several mechanisms through which the stress response precipitates injury have been proposed, including: (a) narrowed peripheral vision, (b) impaired attention, and (c) increased muscle tension. Compromised immune functioning, reduced physical resilience, and increased sensitivity to pain are other possible stress-related consequences that may contribute to sport injury occurrence.

To illustrate how an athlete might sustain an injury in the context of the model shown in Figure 8.1, consider the example of an athlete who tends to get anxious before competing (high competitive trait anxiety), who has experienced a bitter breakup of a romantic relationship in the past few months (history of stressors), and who is playing for a new team in a new city, far away from the athlete's family and friends (low social support). While participating in an important game (potentially stressful sport situation), the athlete thinks about the magnitude of the competition and feels the pressure (cognitive appraisal), experiencing narrowing of peripheral vision, distracting thoughts, and muscle tension. Due to the confluence of psychosocial risk factors, the athlete is "blind-sided" in an ordinarily avoidable collision with an opponent during the game and incurs an injury resulting from the contact with the other player and subsequent fall to the ground.

Preventive interventions

Typical approaches to sport injury prevention involve issuing protective equipment and apparel, maintaining safe facilities for practice and competition, and enhancing the physical preparedness of athletes (e.g., strength, flexibility, endurance) through training. The well-documented links between psychological factors and sport injury occurrence, however, suggest that psychological interventions may also contribute to the prevention of sport injuries. Extrapolating from the model depicted in Figure 8.1, interventions targeting components of the stress response—namely

cognitive appraisals and attentional/physiological changes—should reduce athletes' susceptibility to injury. Consistent with this expectation, stress management interventions have been found effective in decreasing the occurrence of sport injury. Although without empirical support, interventions directed at boosting the social support of athletes would also be expected to lower the injury rate.

Common aspects of stress management programs that have been used to reduce the risk of sustaining sport injuries include cognitive restructuring (which involves learning to recognize and modify counterproductive thoughts), imagery, and relaxation, each of which can have a salubrious effect on the response of athletes to potentially stressful situations. It is noteworthy that the components of stress management interventions overlap with the frequently used sport psychology methods discussed in Chapter 1. This overlap allows for the possibility of athletes to participate in psychological training that may simultaneously enhance their sport performance and decrease their likelihood of becoming injured. Combining psychologically based injury prevention efforts with more physically oriented approaches offers the potential of providing athletes with comprehensive means of minimizing their chances of injury. In circumstances where resources are limited, intervening psychologically only with those athletes whose psychological data suggest that they are at greatest risk for injury may be a valid option.

Injury rehabilitation

When athletes sustain injuries, the immediate focus is generally on physical dimensions of the injuries, such as the location, magnitude, and ramifications of the damage to body tissues. Nevertheless, from the occurrence of sport injuries onward, psychological factors are an integral part of the rehabilitation process. For example, the pain and loss of physical functioning commonly experienced by athletes upon sustaining an injury have strong psychological components. Pain is essentially a psychophysical phenomenon, and a loss of functioning can be defined in terms of

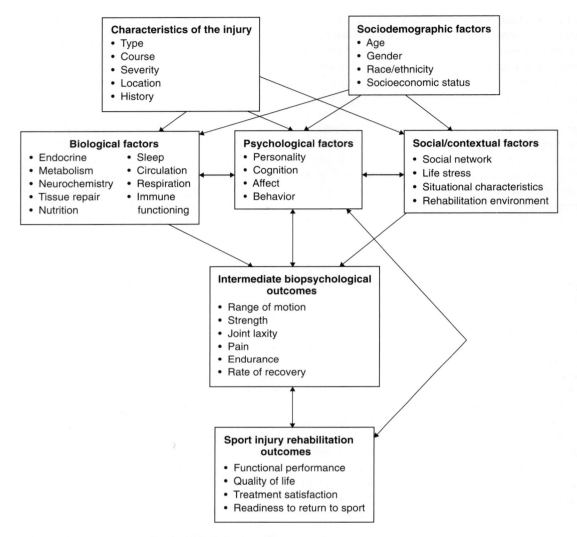

Figure 8.2. A biopsychosocial model of sport injury. *Source*: Brewer, B.W., Andersen, M.B. & Van Raalte, J.L. (2002) Psychological aspects of sport injury rehabilitation: toward a biopsychosocial approach. In D.L. Mostofsky & L.D. Zaichkowsky (eds.) *Medical and Psychological Aspects of Sport and Exercise*, pp. 41–54. Fitness Information Technology, Morgantown. Reprinted with permission

behaviors in which athletes are unable to engage. Not only has a wide variety of psychological effects of sport injury been documented, but psychological factors have been shown to affect the outcome of sport injury rehabilitation.

The biopsychosocial model presented in Figure 8.2 offers a framework for understanding the role of psychological factors in the rehabilitation of sport injuries. In this model, psychological factors

such as personality, cognition (i.e., thinking), affect (i.e., emotions), and behavior are thought to be influenced by both the characteristics of the injury itself and the demographic characteristics of the person sustaining the injury. The emotional responses of a young athlete with a severe, acute injury, for example, might differ dramatically from those of an older athlete with a mild, chronic injury. According to the model, psychological factors affect and are affected by biological factors (e.g., tissue repair, circulation), social factors (e.g., social network, life stress), intermediate biopsychological outcomes (e.g., range of motion, strength, pain), and rehabilitation outcomes (e.g., functional performance, readiness to return to sport). Of particular note, the outcomes on which the success of rehabilitation is largely judged are themselves predominantly psychological or behavioral. Although the physical state of athletes helps to establish a potential of what the athletes are able to accomplish, it is generally what the athletes actually accomplish in the form of behavior (i.e., sport performance) that ultimately determines the outcome of rehabilitation.

Psychological responses to sport injury

As indicated in the biopsychosocial model, sport injury is a stressor that has ramifications for the biological, psychological, and social functioning of athletes. Although their focus is primarily on the biological effects of sport injury, sports medicine practitioners have long been aware of the psychological consequences of sport injury. Initial attempts to describe the psychological responses of athletes to injury borrowed heavily from models of grief and loss, noting parallels between patients with terminal illnesses and athletes with injury in terms of their psychological reactions. With injury prompting a presumed loss of an aspect of the self, athletes were thought to proceed through a sequential series of stages (e.g., denial, anger, bargaining, depression, acceptance) after becoming injured. Unfortunately, research did not support such a characterization of athletes' responses to sport injury. Some athletes *do* exhibit components of a grief reaction after sustaining an injury and athletes generally *do* display more favorable psychological responses with the passage of time following injury, but the notion of a predictable, stage-like sequence of responses that is consistent across athletes simply has not stood up to scientific scrutiny. Instead, the cognitive, emotional, and behavioral reactions of athletes to injury vary considerably and appear to be influenced by a variety of characteristics of the individuals involved and the situations in which they find themselves.

Cognitive responses

The way in which athletes cognitively appraise or interpret their injuries contribute substantially to their psychological adjustment to the challenges posed by the injuries. Injuries perceived as threatening to one's sense of self- and well-being are likely to produce more adverse psychological consequences than injuries construed as neutral, benign, or, in rare cases, beneficial occurrences. Differences in cognitive appraisals help explain the diversity of psychological reactions to the injury exhibited by athletes. For example, athletes who perceive their injuries as resulting in the loss of a self-defining activity are more likely to experience devastating emotional reactions (e.g., depression) than athletes who interpret their injuries as means of escaping the pressures of unwanted sport involvement (and consequently experience thinly disguised feelings of liberation and relief).

Among the common cognitive responses to sport injury are (a) decreased self-esteem; (b) attributional activity; and (c) use of coping strategies. Following injury, athletes tend to experience a drop in evaluations of their self-worth. They readily make attributions regarding the cause(s) of their injuries, some involving factors internal to themselves (e.g., somatic weakness, overtraining) and some pertaining to factors external to themselves (e.g., field conditions, collision with an opponent). In an attempt to cope with the challenges presented by their injuries, athletes deploy a variety of cognitive strategies, such as accepting their injuries, focusing on their rehabilitation tasks, and thinking positive thoughts. Athletes' cognitive responses to injury seem to vary across persons and situations. For example, athletes who are psychologically invested in playing sport professionally are especially likely to experience low self-esteem following career-ending injuries. Further, athletes' self-confidence is likely to wax and wane over the course of rehabilitation, with confidence generally higher at the beginning of rehabilitation and upon achieving recovery than during the rehabilitation process.

Emotional responses

The psychological toll of sport injury is perhaps most evident in the realm of emotions. Among the more common emotions experienced by athletes with injuries are anger, confusion, depression, fear, and frustration. In general, negative emotions tend to increase immediately following injury and decrease over the first month post-injury, presumably as athletes adjust to their conditions and recover health and function. Emotional disturbance may persist, however, when the athletes have severe injuries or encounter obstacles in the recovery progress. In approximately 5–24% of athletes with injuries, the levels of emotional disturbance are clinically meaningful and may warrant the attention of a mental health practitioner. Unfortunately, such emotional distress is not easily recognized by sports medicine professionals and may go undetected.

Several risk factors for emotional distress following sport injury have been identified. Young athletes and athletes who are strongly invested in the athlete role as a source of self-worth tend to experience higher levels of emotional disturbance than those who are older and for whom being an athlete is a less central or exclusive aspect of who they are as a person. Athletes tend to experience greater emotional disturbance when their injuries are severe or long-lasting and when their recovery progress has been slowed. Hardy athletes and those who are satisfied with the social support they are receiving from others tend to experience low levels of emotional disturbance following injury. The timing of injuries in the competitive sport season also seems to play a role in the magnitude of emotional disturbance, as injuries that preclude training for or participation in important events may elicit especially strong emotional reactions.

Behavioral responses

The ways in which athletes respond behaviorally to injury are closely tied to their cognitive and emotional reactions. For example, when athletes cope cognitively with their injury situation by focusing their attention on the tasks of their rehabilitation program, their behavior may be characterized by information-seeking and vigorous pursuit of rehabilitation activities. Similarly, in rare cases where the levels of emotional disturbance in response to injury are extreme, suicidal behavior may result. Although some athletes may seek out social support from others for assistance in dealing with their injuries, other athletes may choose to withdraw socially and attempt to cope with their situation on their own.

The extent to which athletes adhere to prescribed sport injury rehabilitation programs is the post-injury behavior that has received the most attention from researchers. The nature of adherence behavior depends primarily on the specific characteristics of the rehabilitation program such as its location (e.g., home-based, clinic-based) and activity components (e.g., completing exercises, taking medications, limiting sport involvement, receiving therapeutic modalities). Depending on how adherence is measured, rates of adherence to sport injury rehabilitation programs vary considerably, ranging from 40 to 143% (the latter figure due to *over*adherence) in research studies. Higher adherence rates are found when adherence is measured in terms of percentage of rehabilitation sessions attended or percentage of prescribed amount of time spent on rehabilitation activities than when it is assessed by means of classification by level of adherence (e.g., adherent versus non-adherent). Personal characteristics associated with high levels of adherence include being self-motivated, tough-minded, and tolerant of pain. Athletes tend to adhere better to sport injury rehabilitation programs when they believe in the efficacy of the treatment, find the clinical environment comfortable, perceive their rehabilitation appointments as conveniently scheduled, consider their injuries severe, and feel that their rehabilitation efforts are supported by important others. From a cognitive standpoint, adherence rates tend to be higher when athletes ascribe their recovery to factors within their control, view themselves as able to cope with their injuries, set rehabilitation goals, maintain positive self-talk, and use mental imagery. Athletes experiencing emotional disturbance tend to adhere less well to their injury rehabilitation programs than those without such difficulties.

Psychological factors and sport injury rehabilitation outcomes

As suggested by the biopsychosocial model, psychological factors are thought to contribute to both intermediate biopsychological outcomes and sport injury rehabilitation outcomes (which, together, can be considered "outcomes" for the present discussion). For the most part, the relations between psychological factors and sport injury rehabilitation outcomes documented in research studies are *correlational*, which means that the psychological factors cannot yet be considered as direct or even indirect causes of the outcomes. Nevertheless, the relations are suggestive of avenues to investigate in developing interventions for athletes with injuries (and, of course, for conducting further research). For example, although male gender, strong self-identification with the athlete role, and low scores on the personality characteristics of hypochondriasis and hysteria have been linked to faster or better recovery from sport injuries, it cannot be concluded that these factors cause athletes to heal faster or better. Similarly, the finding that higher levels of social support—the lone social/contextual factor that has been linked to sport injury rehabilitation outcomes—are associated with faster recoveries cannot be interpreted as indicating that social support *causes* athletes to recover more rapidly from injury.

Correlational relationships have been documented between many cognitive factors and sport injury rehabilitation outcomes. In general, there seem to be two types of cognition that are associated with recovery from injury—positive thoughts and use of psychological skills. Athletes who demonstrate positive thinking in the form of a positive attitude toward rehabilitation, confidence in their ability to recover, general confidence in themselves, and belief in their ability to affect their recovery tend to heal more quickly than those with more negative thought patterns. Rapid recoveries are also more common among athletes who report using psychological skills such as thought management, healing imagery, and goal setting.

From an emotional standpoint, various forms of psychological distress have been linked to less favorable sport injury rehabilitation outcomes. Athletes who display general mood disturbance or specific negative emotions such as depression, tension, fatigue, fear, frustration, and rehabilitation anxiety tend to recover from their injuries more slowly than those without such emotional difficulties.

Although behaviors such as being physically active, engaging in active coping, and seeking social support have been tied to positive sport injury rehabilitation outcomes, the behavior that has been most frequently associated with recovery from sport injury is adherence to the prescribed rehabilitation program. The link between treatment adherence and rehabilitation outcome seems both obvious and straightforward, but that is not the case. For better adherence to produce a better outcome, it is necessary for the rehabilitation program to be unquestionably effective. If the rehabilitation program is anything less than effective in producing desired treatment outcomes, even complete and total adherence to the program is unlikely to yield the intended results. Moreover, because adherence is generally not the exclusive determinant of rehabilitation outcomes, exemplary levels of adherence to the rehabilitation program may not be sufficient to offset the influence of other biological, psychological, and social/contextual factors thought to play key roles in the recovery process. As a consequence, some athletes may heal rapidly despite adhering poorly to their rehabilitation program, whereas other athletes may recover slowly even though they do all that is asked of them by the rehabilitation professionals supervising their care.

The nature of the relationships between psychological factors and sport injury rehabilitation outcomes is not fully understood. Although it is plausible that rehabilitation adherence could have a direct impact on recovery from sport injury (by improving strength, flexibility, endurance, etc.), it is likely that the effects of most of the psychological factors correlated with sport injury rehabilitation outcomes—if they have an effect—are indirect, influencing outcomes through intermediary variables more closely related to indices of injury recovery. For example, emotional disturbance may affect immune functioning, which, in turn, may influence tissue repair and other aspects of healing. Similarly, adopting a positive attitude toward rehabilitation, believing that one can influence rehabilitation outcomes, and feeling supported by family members and friends may help to facilitate adherence to the rehabilitation program, which, again, may contribute to enhanced readiness to return to sport participation, better quality of life, improved satisfaction with the course of treatment, and elevated performance of functional sport tasks.

Psychological interventions to enhance rehabilitation

As knowledge of the relevance of psychological factors to sport injury rehabilitation outcomes has grown, psychological interventions have been increasingly applied to enhance the rehabilitation of athletes with injuries. The effectiveness of several interventions has been documented in experimental studies, which allow inferences to be made about the causal role of psychological factors in sport injury rehabilitation. Nevertheless, as with the psychological factors for which correlational relationships with sport injury rehabilitation outcomes have been established, the exact mechanisms by which psychological interventions influence processes and outcomes in sport injury rehabilitation are not fully understood. Such understanding is not necessary to use and benefit from psychological interventions, but knowing more about the mechanisms of effect will likely contribute to the development and implementation of even more effective interventions. Psychological interventions that have been found effective in experimental investigations include biofeedback, relaxation/imagery, goal setting, self-talk, and treatment packages combining multiple intervention strategies.

Biofeedback is an intervention that involves giving (or "feeding back") physiological information to individuals in an attempt to alter a related physiological process, behavior, or psychological state. Although a wide variety of physiological variables can be assessed in different forms of biofeedback (e.g., blood pressure, heart rate, skin temperature), electromyographic (EMG) activity (i.e., muscle tension) is the physiological parameter that has been used most frequently in the biofeedback given to athletes with injuries. In particular, EMG biofeedback has been administered to assist athletes regain quadriceps strength and range of motion in the knee joint following surgery.

As in other areas of sport psychology practice, although relaxation and imagery are separate interventions with potentially disparate goals, they are often paired in treating athletes with injuries.

Relaxation enables athletes to calm their minds and bodies, thereby facilitating the introduction of mental images. Common imagery themes used in association with sport injury rehabilitation are motivation (e.g., returning successfully to sport participation), healing (e.g., increasing circulation to affected area), and rehearsal of physical skills (e.g., sport or rehabilitation tasks).

In the context of sport injury rehabilitation, goal setting involves generating a set of personal behavioral standards to achieve during rehabilitation. Typically, both short- and long-term rehabilitation goals are established. Appropriate goal targets generally correspond to behaviors over which athletes can exert control, such as the number of repetitions of a particular rehabilitation exercise or the amount of time spent performing a given rehabilitation activity. Reducing injury-related pain and functional impairment are worthy aims of rehabilitation, but are essentially outcomes that are potentially influenced by factors other than the behavior of athletes with injuries and are therefore likely inappropriate targets of goal setting. Progress toward goal completion is monitored and goals are adjusted as necessary, making the targets more or less challenging depending on the level of goal progress. To increase the likelihood of achieving successful completion of goals that have been established, barriers to goal attainment can be identified and strategies to conquer or evade the obstacles can be devised.

In the context of sport injury rehabilitation, positive self-talk is focused on creating an encouraging internal dialog to counteract the discouraging and challenging circumstances in which athletes with injuries find themselves. In positive self-talk interventions, athletes are taught to recognize negative thoughts and replace them with more productive thoughts. By counteracting the negativity, athletes can enhance their attitude and emotional state, improve their motivation to engage in rehabilitation activities, and, ultimately, bolster their rehabilitation progress.

Although discussed separately, the various psychological interventions used to enhance sport injury rehabilitation are often combined into multimodal treatment packages. The interventions are highly complementary. For example, the targets of goal setting can include not only behaviors such as performing rehabilitation exercises and attending physiotherapy sessions but also engaging in rehabilitation-related activities such as imagery and biofeedback, and the content of images and positive self-talk may correspond closely to the rehabilitation goals that the athletes have set. Given their complementary nature, the interventions can be presented to athletes as components of an integrated, comprehensive approach to injury rehabilitation.

Practical considerations

Despite the growing body of research in support of their efficacy, psychological interventions are rarely used in the context of sport injury prevention and rehabilitation. There are several possible reasons for this. First, the scientific studies supporting the use of psychological interventions in the sport injury realm have been published largely in journals read primarily by psychologists or sport psychologists. Sports medicine practitioners, who constitute the front lines in the prevention and treatment of sport injuries, may simply be unaware of the potential utility of psychological interventions in their work. Second, even when those authorized to make decisions about preventive and rehabilitative interventions are aware of and receptive to psychological applications, there can be limitations in the availability and accessibility of professionals with the requisite expertise and qualifications for implementing psychological interventions with athletes. Third, with respect to preventive interventions, coaches are sometimes reluctant to allocate valuable time for programming that addresses problems that are likely (in most sports) to emerge but have not yet developed. The typical low cost and potentially beneficial "side effects" of preventive psychological interventions (e.g., improved ability to cope with life and sport stressors) are arguments against such reluctance. Fourth, regarding psychological intervention with athletes who are already injured, emotional disturbance is not always readily apparent to those treating the injury, so sports medicine practitioners may experience difficulties

in determining which athletes to refer for psychological consultation. Because psychological interventions are potentially useful for many athletes with injury, not just those displaying distress, professionals treating the athletes from a medical perspective can routinely enlist the assistance of a sport psychology consultant (where such an individual is available) as part of a holistic approach to rehabilitation. Such an approach may also serve to minimize any sort of stigma associated with consulting a sport psychology practitioner.

An advantage in implementing psychological interventions for sport injury prevention is that there is generally a good deal of flexibility in terms of when, where, how, and by whom the interventions are delivered. As with any preventive intervention, it is ideal if they are administered before extensive exposure to risk occurs, which, for athletes, is early in the preseason period. Participating in these interventions does not typically involve physical exertion, so they can be planned for blocks of time before, after, or between training sessions. Preventive psychological interventions can be implemented indoors and, depending on the weather and mode of presentation, outdoors in classroom, sport, and other facilities. As they are essentially educational programs, the interventions can be delivered efficiently in both individual and large or small group formats through live and, potentially, multimedia (e.g., Internet) presentation methods. Conceivably, the interventions can be presented to athletes not only by sport psychology consultants, but also by professionals in other disciplines (e.g., coaches, physiotherapists) who are knowledgeable of the curriculum.

Intervening psychologically with athletes after they have been injured can be considerably more complex and challenging than doing so preventively. Although psychological intervention can begin at any time following injury, it can be difficult to determine the exact point at which to intervene, the type of intervention to provide, and the particular professional to deliver the intervention unless a sport psychology consultant is an integral part of the sports medicine treatment team and post-injury psychological evaluation is standard. An initial decision involves whether to intervene proactively or to wait until psychological or other problems have developed before intervening. This decision is influenced by factors such as the sports medicine team's treatment philosophy and the availability of professionals to provide psychological intervention. The type of intervention to be implemented is determined primarily by the goals or purpose of the intervention. For example, a different intervention is likely to be selected for an athlete who is experiencing difficulty sleeping as a result of reduced physical activity following injury than for an athlete who is having trouble adhering to the prescribed rehabilitation program. Determining the appropriate practitioner to intervene psychologically is also influenced largely by the reasons for which intervention is sought. When the reasons involve concerns regarding the mental health of the athlete in question, a professional with expertise in assessing and treating clinical issues should be consulted. With the permission of the athlete, some interventions, such as goal setting, imagery, and biofeedback, can be optimized through consultation and coordination with the physiotherapist or other sports medicine practitioner overseeing the care of the athlete. Regardless of the psychological interventions selected or the professionals chosen to implement the interventions, it is important that the interventions are not be viewed as "extra" or "additional" by the athletes. Despite the common perception that athletes with injuries have more "time on their hands," they often have *less* available time than they would when uninjured due to ongoing team commitments (e.g., attending practice sessions), treatment obligations, and cross-training activities (where feasible). Presenting psychological interventions as just another modality within the overall treatment program can enhance the acceptability of the interventions to the athletes. Careful consideration of the timing, nature, providers, and framing of psychological interventions can help to ensure that the interests of athletes with injuries are best served.

CASE STUDIES

CASE STUDY 1

Athletes

The athletes were members of a national women's Under 21 football (soccer) team. Many of the players were drawn from the professional ranks, and the core of the team had been playing together internationally since their tenure on the Under 19 squad 2 years earlier. Based on its performance over the previous year, the team appeared to be in strong contention for a berth in the upcoming Olympic Games.

Reason for consultancy

Well aware of the on-field success of several other prominent teams in the sport that had employed a sport psychology consultant, the team's head coach sought to gain a competitive edge by enlisting the services of a sport psychologist. Outside of general performance enhancement, the coach did not have any particular agenda when she contacted the sport psychology consultant available to her through the national governing body.

Background

The team had achieved a fairly consistent level of success in international competition. The coach had a reputation for implementing a rigorous, but not excessive training regime. Despite their physical preparation, the players had experienced an unusually high injury rate over the past 2 years, with several team members incurring season-ending injuries.

Professional assessment

As a prelude to working with the team, the sport psychology consultant conducted lengthy interviews with the head coach, assistant coaches, and team captains to find out how she could best serve the team. These discussions revealed no major team chemistry issues and no glaring psychological weaknesses at the team level. The coaches and captains cited the ongoing challenges of travel, training, and competition as the main issues confronting the team.

Intervention

In the absence of any pressing issues requiring immediate attention, the sport psychology consultant proposed a series of introductory workshops focusing on basic psychological skills of potential utility to elite athletes. In addition to the educational function of the workshops, they were designed to introduce the sport psychologist to the team and pave the way for future individual consultations. Featuring interactive group presentations on topics such as cognitive restructuring, imagery, and relaxation; the intervention was essentially a cognitive-behavioral stress management intervention, as the consultant emphasized ways in which the psychological skills could be used inside and outside of the sport context to manage competitive and life stress. In the workshops, the athletes identified common sources of stress that they encountered and practiced using their newly acquired psychological skills to cope with the stressors.

CASE STUDIES (Continued)

Outcome

Given the initial high performance level of the team and the lack of obvious psychological deficiencies at the team level, effects of the intervention on competitive performance were not immediately evident. The team members, however, were receptive to the intervention, reporting that they found the sessions "relaxing," enjoyed the team-oriented time off the pitch, and appreciated the engaging presentational style of the sport psychology consultant. Of particular note, in marked contrast to previous years, the team members sustained no major injuries and only a few minor injuries over the course of the competitive season. On the basis of the apparent injury-reducing effect of and the team's receptivity to the intervention, the head coach retained the services of the consultant up to and throughout the Olympic Games.

CASE STUDY 2

Athlete

Adam was a 24-year-old male triathlete ranked in the bottom half of the top ten competitors in his country. He had sufficient financial support to train full-time for his sport. In the middle of the competitive season of a non-Olympic year and after 8 weeks of progressively worsening leg pain, Adam had a bone scan and was diagnosed with a femoral stress fracture in his right leg. The injury prevented him from participating in the remaining events of the season.

Reason for consultancy

Adam was referred by his physiotherapist to a clinically trained sport psychologist ostensibly for "adjunctive mental training to accompany the rehabilitation program." In actuality, the physiotherapist was concerned about apparent emotional disturbance, episodes of treatment non-adherence, and slower than expected progress through rehabilitation.

Background

Although swimming was his original discipline, Adam had been training for all three triathlon disciplines and participating in triathlons since age 17. He was regarded as a hard worker among his peers, even by the sport's lofty standards. In addition to running, swimming, and cycling, Adam was involved regularly in a strength and plyometric training program. Approximately 10 weeks prior to receiving his stress fracture diagnosis, Adam began experiencing occasional discomfort in his lower thigh. When the problem did not dissipate over the next few weeks, he sought treatment. The physiotherapist gave Adam a preliminary diagnosis of iliotibial band syndrome and prescribed cryotherapy, an anti-inflammatory medication, and a brief stretching routine. Adam followed the prescribed treatment religiously while maintaining his intensive training and competition schedule.

The treatment regimen helped Adam to manage the pain, which ebbed and flowed as a function of the particular training activities of the day. His discomfort gradually worsened until

he could no longer maintain his running form and began experiencing compensatory problems in his left leg. An X-ray was negative, so Adam kept on training and competing. Eventually, when Adam could not walk without experiencing significant discomfort, a bone scan was prescribed. The scan was positive, revealing a stress fracture in the lower third of his right femur. Initially, Adam was relieved to find out what his problem was, that it wasn't "all in his head," but he quickly realized that his training would be curtailed dramatically and he would not be able to finish the competitive season due to the prescribed 8-week period of rest (with respect to running). He continued swimming and strength training as part of a "no impact" training program, but was deeply disappointed with the 2 kg weight gain he incurred in the first month of his rehabilitation. Counter to his doctor's instructions, Adam began a premature return to cycling that resulted in a re-aggravation of his symptoms and set back his healing several weeks. Adam became frustrated and despondent about his regression. His physiotherapist noticed the change in Adam's demeanor and discussed with Adam the possibility of working with a sport psychologist to "focus his approach to rehabilitation in a positive direction."

Intervention

In response to the physiotherapist's constructive referral strategy, Adam proclaimed that he would "do anything" to hasten his recovery and agreed to meet with the sport psychology consultant. After an initial interview in which Adam described the rehabilitation situation from his perspective, the sport psychologist concluded that although Adam was clearly upset, his distress was focused specifically on his injury problem and did not likely constitute a clinical disorder. Two interrelated issues were identified as problematic—Adam's desire to resume various aspects of his training program before medically indicated and his feeling that he was "not doing enough" to speed his healing. To address the first issue, the sport psychologist helped Adam view his attempts to "test" his leg's ability to withstand cycling before his doctor had consented for him to do so as acting in a counterproductive and undisciplined manner. Discipline was clearly something that Adam valued and by reframing his refraining from "testing" his leg as indicative of mental strength, he was able to talk himself away from the temptation to go against his doctor's wishes. Given Adam's propensity for hard work, the sport psychology consultant addressed the second issue by getting Adam involved in a program of relaxation and guided imagery that included both healing and sport performance images. This intervention was recommended to give Adam a sense of control over his recovery, help him manage the stresses of rehabilitation, and provide him with a way to keep his sport skills salient in his mind.

Outcome

Although the relaxation portion of the intervention did not come naturally to Adam, he was able to generate a set of vivid healing and sport performance images over the course of rehabilitation. He adhered fully to the rehabilitation program and expressed pride at being able to show the discipline necessary to avoid returning prematurely to his sport activities. Due to his early mishaps, Adam took approximately 2 weeks longer than originally anticipated to recover and resume, gradually, his standard training program. He still exhibited a tendency toward overtraining, but seemed better able to step back, discern the messages he was receiving from his body, and reduce his training load for a day or two until he felt better. Once recovered, Adam stopped using healing imagery, but continued to practice sport performance imagery on a regular basis to "get the most" out of his mind and body.

Further reading

Brewer, B.W. (2007) Psychology of sport injury rehabilitation. In G. Tenenbaum & R.C. Eklund (eds.) *Handbook of Sport Psychology*, 3rd Edn, pp. 404–424. Wiley, New York.

Johnson, U. (2007) Psychosocial antecedents of sport injury, prevention, and intervention: an overview of theoretical approaches and empirical findings. *International Journal of Sport and Exercise Psychology* **5**, 352–369.

Pargman, D. (ed.) (2007) *Psychological Bases of Sport Injuries*, 3rd Edn. Fitness Information Technology, Morgantown.

Williams, J.M., Andersen, M.B. (2007) Psychosocial antecedents of sport injury and interventions for risk reduction. In G. Tenenbaum & R.C. Eklund (eds.) *Handbook of Sport Psychology*, 3rd Edn, pp. 379–403. Wiley, New York.

Chapter 9
Clinical issues

Britton W. Brewer

Department of Psychology, Springfield College, Springfield, MA, USA

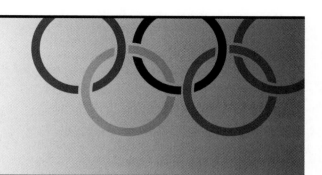

Introduction

Despite the pioneering endeavors of Norman Triplett, Coleman Griffith, and others in applying psychology to sport performance, for many years the traditional conceptualization of psychologists in the context of sport was as mental health providers. Over the past few decades, the role of psychologists in sport has expanded considerably, particularly with respect to the delivery of performance enhancement services to teams and individual athletes. Nevertheless, addressing clinical concerns with athletes has remained an important, albeit less visible, aspect of sport psychology service delivery.

The need for athletes to receive attention from a clinical practitioner frequently, but not always, coincides with the presence of diagnosable psychopathology. In general, clinical issues emerge when athletes encounter substantial psychological distress, behave in a manner that deviates from the prevailing norms of the social and cultural context in which they live, experience impairment in their ability to carry out tasks of daily living, or constitute a danger to themselves or other people. Although the common conception of athletes is one of the high-functioning individuals, athletes are nonetheless susceptible to the same sorts of psychological problems encountered by the general population. Indeed, even though involvement in vigorous

Sport Psychology. 1st edition. Edited by Britton Brewer.
Published 2009 by Blackwell Publishing.
ISBN 978-1-4051-7363-6.

physical activity characteristic of sport participation is often associated with favorable mental health outcomes, athletes are exposed to situational and environmental pressures that can heighten their vulnerability to certain forms of psychopathology. The purpose of this chapter is to review some of the mental disorders commonly experienced by athletes and discuss matters specific to the diagnosis, referral, and treatment of athletes with issues warranting the attention of a clinical practitioner.

Psychopathology in sport

There are few epidemiological data available on which to base estimates of the prevalence of mental disorders among athletes. Although the demands of competitive sport is likely to preclude the involvement of a large number of individuals with the most severe forms of psychopathology, athletes experiencing a wide variety of mental disorders have been documented in case studies and anecdotal reports. Among the forms of psychopathology that have been identified in association with top level athletes are anorexia nervosa, attention-deficit hyperactivity disorder (ADHD), bipolar disorder, body dysmorphic disorder, borderline personality disorder, bulimia nervosa, conversion disorder, major depressive disorder, narcissistic personality disorder, obsessive compulsive disorder, panic disorder, seasonal affective disorder, schizoaffective disorder, and Tourette's disorder. Surveys of clinical practitioners who work with athletes suggest that anxiety, depression, eating disorders, and substance-related disorders are the most common types of psychopathology for which athletes receive treatment.

Anxiety

Anxiety is a normal part of everyday life. People commonly encounter situations in which they experience one or more of the typical symptoms of anxiety, including those in the cognitive (e.g., worries), emotional (e.g., feelings of nervousness), behavioral (e.g., pacing), and physiological (e.g., muscle tension) domains. Most of the anxiety experienced by athletes, even that which occurs prior to competition and is of sufficient magnitude to have an adverse effect on sport performance, is subclinical and can be dealt with through performance enhancement interventions (see Chapter 4).

In some cases, however, the anxiety experienced by athletes is severe enough or long enough in duration that it causes athletes discomfort or impairs their ability to perform tasks of daily living. In instances such as the chronic state of unrealistic and excessive worry characteristic of generalized anxiety disorder or the full-blown episodes of intense anxiety symptoms that occur as part of panic disorder, athletes warrant the attention of a clinical practitioner for the purposes of assessment, diagnosis, and treatment of their pathological condition. Unfortunately, prevalence rates for anxiety disorders in athletes are not available. Although physical activity such as that routinely engaged in by athletes can help reduce anxiety; there is no reason to believe that the prevalence of anxiety disorders for athletes differs substantially from the prevalence for the general population.

An example of a sport-specific manifestation of an anxiety disorder is what has been labeled as a "sport performance phobia," in which the anxiety of athletes is focused on a particular task or element of their overall sport performance. Case illustrations of this condition include gymnasts and divers who balk at performing specific moves or dives that they have accomplished in the past and currently possess the requisite skills to achieve, a tennis player who fears approaching the net and avoids doing so while playing, and a baseball catcher who, despite possessing the ability to throw

the ball to second base, cannot toss the ball back to the pitcher. Extreme anxiety reactions such as these and those associated with obsessive-compulsive disorder and post-traumatic stress disorder should be addressed by clinically trained practitioners.

Depression

As with anxiety disorders, there are few epidemiological data on the prevalence of depressive disorders among competitive athletes. Preliminary surveys conducted with competitive athlete samples suggest that approximately one in five athletes experiences depressive symptoms of the magnitude observed in individuals with clinical depression. The extent to which the symptoms reflect depressive disorders (e.g., major depressive disorder, dysthymic disorder, seasonal affective disorder) as opposed to adjustment reactions to pain, injury, deselection, chronic competitive failure, and other adverse sport and non-sport life circumstances is not known. Adjustment disorder with depressed mood involves experiencing symptoms of major depression (e.g., sadness, worthlessness, appetite disturbance, sleep disruption, anger, irritability, guilt, fatigue, apathy, concentration difficulties) that are triggered by a specific stressful event or situation, last less than 6 months, and dissipate soon after the circumstances that precipitated the symptoms are resolved. In rare (but sometimes widely publicized) instances, athletes displaying depressive symptoms may attempt or commit suicide. Consequently, when athletes exhibit symptoms of depression that go beyond transitory feelings of sadness or disappointment, regardless of whether they are depressive disorders or adjustment reactions, the attention of a clinical practitioner is warranted.

Similar to the way in which exercise can reduce anxiety, physical activity can decrease both depressed mood and clinical depression. Nevertheless, excessive physical training can, in some cases, produce symptoms that mimic those of both depression and chronic fatigue syndrome. Athletes, who develop the condition known as staleness in response to high-volume training, encounter a decrement in sport performance along with mood, sleep, and appetite disturbances. When such circumstances arise, it is important for athletes to back off on their training and for practitioners to evaluate the athletes carefully to verify the source of the symptoms and check if the athletes are experiencing a depressive disorder instead of or in addition to the apparent staleness.

Eating disorders

One of the few areas of psychopathology where substantial epidemiological data are available is eating disorders. Estimates of the prevalence of eating disorders among competitive athletes have varied widely, depending largely on the methods and measures used to determine the estimates. When stringent diagnostic criteria are applied, the prevalence rates for anorexia nervosa and bulimia nervosa in athletes approximate those for the general population (0.5–1.0% and 1.0–3.0%, respectively, with rates roughly 10 times higher for women than for men). For subclinical eating disorders, however, where eating behavior is problematic but not to the extent that diagnostic criteria are fully satisfied, prevalence rates are much higher than those for diagnosable conditions and may be even higher for athletes than non-athletes. In addition, female athletes are susceptible to the *female athlete triad*, which refers to disordered eating, menstrual dysfunction (e.g., amenorrhea, oligomenorrhea), and low bone mass (i.e., osteoporosis, osteopenia), a combination that places women at an elevated risk for musculoskeletal injury (e.g., stress fractures).

It is widely accepted that biological, psychological, and social factors contribute to the development of disordered eating in the general population. There are several additional factors specific to the sport environment that influence the occurrence of eating disturbances in athletes. Competitors in esthetic sports (e.g., figure skating, gymnastics) and some endurance sports (e.g., distance running) may acquire the perception that losing weight will enhance their performance. To the extent that athletes deviate (or perceive themselves as deviating) from the lean stereotype associated with their sport, they may experience pressure to engage in disordered eating in an attempt to lose weight. Although the methods that athletes sometimes use to lose weight (e.g., fasting, dieting, vomiting, using laxatives) may not be

endorsed explicitly, athletes may find their weight loss efforts supported by coaches and others in the sport system, reinforcing the acceptability of pathogenic eating behavior and, more generally, of compromising one's health in the pursuit of enhanced sport performance. Similarly, athletes may obtain support in the sport environment for displaying characteristics that overlap with salient aspects of disordered eating, such as attempting to achieve perfection, engaging in excessive physical activity, and ignoring pain or discomfort.

Treatment of clinical eating disorders clearly warrants the involvement of a mental health practitioner. Depending on symptom severity, the presence of subclinical disordered eating may also merit professional attention. Given the potential influence of the sport environment on the eating behavior of athletes, recommendations for prevention of eating disorders in athletes include weighing athletes only when necessary for medical reasons, formulating individualized training programs that focus on health rather than weight, and minimizing pressures to lose weight or change body size. Although athletes are not divorced from the societal forces that contribute to the occurrence of eating disorders, coaches are well positioned to initiate these recommendations and foster the development of a climate where healthy eating behavior can flourish in the pursuit of sport performance goals.

Substance-related disorders

As a function of their involvement in competitive sport, athletes can encounter considerable difficulties in association with drug use. In addition to facing the legal, physical, and mental consequences of substance intoxication, abuse, and dependence, athletes are subject to disqualification from sport competition, restriction of their ability to pursue a sport career, and unfavorable publicity. Complicating matters is the fact that athletes may use drugs for both recreational and performance enhancement reasons. Consequently, some substances that are legal for use by the general population are banned for competitors in certain sports. Although the frequency of drug testing varies across sports and levels of competition, it is safe to say that, in general, the drug use of athletes is scrutinized to a greater degree than that of their non-athlete peers.

In contrast with the images of a healthy lifestyle that are often associated with involvement in sport and physical activity, epidemiological data from North America suggest that despite restricting their consumption of alcohol during the competitive season, high school and college athletes use alcohol, become intoxicated with alcohol, and engage in alcohol-drinking binges more than non-athletes. Recreational use of other substances, particularly marijuana, has also been documented in competitive athletes. In addition to using drugs for recreational purposes, some athletes turn to banned substances for reasons of performance enhancement. Among the performance enhancing functions of these substances are increasing muscle strength and size (e.g., anabolic steroids), improving the oxygen-carrying capacity of the blood (e.g., erythropoietin), accelerating recovery and healing (e.g., human growth hormone), decreasing pain (e.g., morphine, oxycontin), increasing energy (e.g., amphetamines), decreasing physiological arousal (e.g., beta-blockers), and controlling weight (e.g., diuretics). Information on the prevalence of the use of banned substances by competitive athletes is, understandably, limited.

Various physical, psychological, and social factors contribute to drug use by athletes. The factors parallel those influencing the drug use of the general public, but include additional contributors that are unique to involvement in competitive sport. For example, physical effects such as increased energy, heightened alertness, improved relaxation, and pain reduction can affect the substance-using behavior of anyone, but take on added meaning in the context of sport performance enhancement. Similarly, psychological factors such as boredom, desire to escape unpleasant emotions, low self-confidence, and personal problems may precipitate drug use both inside and outside of the sport environment. In terms of social contributors, the drug use of athletes can be affected by pressure from their athlete and non-athlete peers alike, with the *perceived* use of banned substances by competitors especially salient in the choice to take performance-enhancing drugs.

For substance use conditions involving intoxication, abuse, or dependence (the latter two of which involve distress or impaired functioning over an extended period of time), athletes should be referred to a specialist for treatment. Depending on the nature and severity of the problem, athletes are likely to receive inpatient or outpatient treatment involving detoxification, some form of retraining (e.g., therapy, coping skills development), and follow-up (e.g., status monitoring, peer support, additional retraining). Efforts directed at preventing drug use by athletes typically involve the implementation of strategies such as deterrence (primarily through drug testing and associated penalties for use of banned substances), education about the causes and consequences of drug use, and training in coping, drug refusal, and/or life skills. Appeals based primarily on fear have not generally proven successful in the prevention of drug use in sport.

Various disorders

Several other clinical conditions have particular relevance for competitive athletes: muscle dysmorphia, pathological gambling, and concussion. Muscle dysmorphia is a proposed subtype of body dysmorphic disorder, a somatoform diagnosis involving preoccupation with an imagined appearance deficit that produces impairment and/or distress. In the instance of muscle dysmorphia, which is anecdotally considered common among male weightlifters and bodybuilders, the pathological preoccupation is with insufficient leanness and muscularity. Behavioral responses are likely to involve dieting, weightlifting, and other means of remedying the perceived deficit. Although it is clear that muscle dysmorphia is a condition that warrants the attention of a clinical practitioner, empirically supported methods for treating the disorder have not been developed.

Gambling in the forms of betting on sporting events, online gambling, casino gaming, and playing cards or other games of chance for money is common in many societies around the world. The behavior becomes pathological when people exhibit five or more symptoms such as being preoccupied with gambling, requiring increasingly larger or more frequent wagering to produce the same magnitude of positive feelings from gambling, gambling to improve one's mood or escape negative emotions, attempting to win back losses through further gambling, lying about one's degree of involvement with gambling, trying unsuccessfully to curb one's gambling, and violating the law to acquire funds for gambling. Gambling has ramifications not only for the personal adjustment of athletes, but also for their sport participation eligibility and, potentially, for the integrity of the sports in which they participate. Although high-profile athletes in a variety of sports have experienced well-publicized difficulties with gambling, information regarding the prevalence, etiology, and treatment of pathological gambling among athletes is lacking. It is clear, however, that treatment of an impulse control disorder such as this should be performed by a mental health professional.

Athletes participating in contact and collision sports (e.g., football, ice hockey) and certain self-paced sports (e.g., mountain biking, skiing, snowboarding) are at an elevated risk for sustaining a concussion, an injury that occurs when the brain is shaken within the skull. Concussions produce an array of symptoms that is not uniform across individuals and includes such responses as amnesia, disorientation, emotional disturbance (e.g., depression, irritability), fatigue, headache, loss of consciousness, nausea, and sleep disturbance. The rate of symptom resolution after concussion is highly variable, both across and within individuals across symptoms. Post-concussive symptoms may resolve quickly (i.e., within a few days) for some athletes, but may linger for months for other athletes. Similarly, for a given athlete, although most symptoms may remit rapidly, other symptoms (e.g., cognitive impairment, headache) may persist. Contemporary approaches to sport-related concussion involve obtaining pre-season baseline measurements of neurocognitive factors (e.g., attention, learning, memory) before implementing a more extensive post-concussive management protocol. Upon sustaining a concussion, athletes typically will be examined medically to rule out more serious injury, educated about the consequences of concussion, prescribed rest (both physical and mental), and prevented from resuming sport participation until they match their baseline neurocognitive performance and demonstrate the ability to exert themselves physically without experiencing a return of their symptoms.

Culture and other demographic influences on athlete psychopathology

Demographic factors can play a key role in how athletes experience and express psychological problems as well as how those problems are interpreted and viewed by athletes and others. Culture is an especially salient influence on athlete psychopathology. For example, there is cross-cultural variation in the expression of emotion, a key element of many clinical conditions. Athletes from some cultural backgrounds exhibit outwardly a wide range of emotions, whereas athletes from other cultures are more reserved in their emotional expression. Similarly, cultures vary in the extent to which seeking help for psychological disorders is considered acceptable, the amount of stigma associated with psychological problems, and the types of practitioners deemed appropriate to treat psychological difficulties. Such variability affects the likelihood of athletes in distress attempting to gain assistance and from whom. In the extreme, there are some culture-bound syndromes that occur predominantly or exclusively within specific cultural groups (e.g., amok, koro) and are explained and treated in accord with local customs.

The psychopathology of athletes is influenced not only by the culture of their nation, region, or ethnic group, but also by the culture of sport, which can transcend national, regional, and ethnic boundaries. Involvement in sport often comes with a set of values, traditions, and behavioral expectations that can differ markedly from those of the general public and to which athletes are socialized from an early age through their exposure to and interactions with coaches, fellow athletes, spectators, and the media. Athletes may acquire attributes that, depending on the task demands of the specific sport in which they are involved, may be quite adaptive on the playing field (e.g., toughness, aggressiveness, detachment, lack of social conformity), but, if taken to an extreme outside of sport, may be indicative of psychopathology. Likewise, although the single-minded devotion to sport that athletes are often encouraged to adopt can have a facilitative effect on the athletes' motivation to train and compete, it can also foster the development of a narrow self-identity that can leave athletes susceptible to psychological disturbance when they experience events that threaten their self-identity (e.g., deselection, injury, sport career termination).

Living within the culture of sport can expose athletes to stressors that can contribute to the onset of psychological problems. Competition with teammates for playing time, injury, pain, pressure from coaches, restricted social interaction, and constant scrutiny from the media both inside and outside the sport environment are among the sport-related situations that can contribute to a variety of psychological reactions, including anxiety, depression, and paranoia. Compounding matters is that the social support provided to athletes, which can serve as a buffer against the stressful events they encounter, is often contingent on successful sport performance. Athletes not performing up to the expectations of their coaches or the sport administrators sometimes find that the supportive social interactions to which they had become accustomed are withdrawn just when they need them the most. Even when things are going well for athletes in terms of performance, the social support they receive may come in the form of coddling and adulation, both of which may contribute to narcissism and other personality problems.

In addition to culture, gender and age are demographic factors of particular relevance to athlete psychopathology. With respect to gender, substantial differences between men and women in prevalence rates are evident for some clinical conditions. In general, women are more likely to have "emotional" disorders (e.g., major depression), whereas men are at greater risk for "behavioral" disorders (e.g., antisocial personality disorder). However, tendencies are by no means universal across cultures and although some of the gender differences in prevalence can be attributed to biology, it is likely that the process by which men and women learn expected masculine and feminine attitudes and behaviors (i.e., gender

socialization) and the differential life experiences of men and women also contribute strongly to the prevalence differences. For example, there is evidence that the occurrence of anorexia nervosa and bulimia nervosa, conditions for which women athletes are at substantially greater risk than men athletes, is affected in part by societal definitions of attractiveness.

As with gender, prevalence rates for certain mental disorders vary as a function of age. Although many disorders can affect athletes at any point in the life cycle, some conditions are more likely to occur at specific points of the age spectrum. Some sleep disorders (e.g., sleepwalking disorder, nightmare disorder), tend to resolve by late childhood. Other disorders, however, such as bipolar disorder (i.e., manic depression) and bulimia nervosa commonly have onsets in late adolescence or early adulthood. Age serves as a proxy for developmental milestones in physical (e.g., puberty), psychological, and social (e.g., leaving home) functioning, any and all of which can affect the manifestation of clinical conditions by athletes. Consequently, it is essential to put the psychological problems of athletes into an appropriate developmental context, taking into account the age of the athletes when considering the potential causes, course, and consequences of their difficulties.

Addressing clinical issues in sport

Although the nature and circumstances of the clinical issues experienced by athletes vary considerably, there is a fairly standard sequence of events that occurs once athlete psychopathology has been identified. As depicted in Figure 9.1, the sequence involves recognition of the clinical issue, referral to a clinically trained professional, assessment of the athlete's behavior and situation, diagnosis of the athlete's problem, and treatment of the disorder.

Recognition

Before a clinical issue can be addressed, it must first be recognized. The people in the best position to recognize clinical issues in athletes are those who

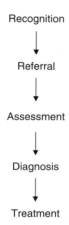

Recognition

↓

Referral

↓

Assessment

↓

Diagnosis

↓

Treatment

Figure 9.1. Typical sequence of events in addressing clinical issues in athletes

have the most contact with the athletes. Beginning with the athletes themselves, these individuals are likely to include teammates, coaches, sports medicine personnel, friends, and family members. Recognizing psychopathology can be both challenging and discomforting for those not trained to do so, it is not necessary for specific disorders to be identified. Instead, it is sufficient to notice when athletes are experiencing distress, deviating from their typical mode of behavior, behaving in such a way that their performance (in sport or other important life domains) suffers substantially, or constituting a danger to themselves or others.

Referral

Once a clinical issue has been identified, the next step is referral to a professional trained to deal with psychopathology. Clinical or counseling psychologists, psychiatrists, and clinical social workers are among the types of professionals most likely to possess the expertise to address clinical issues in athletes. The simplest form of referral is self-referral, when athletes notice their problems on their own and seek professional assistance either directly or through intermediaries (e.g., coaches, sports medicine practitioners). Referrals generated by people other than the affected athletes themselves are especially delicate. Optimally,

the individuals making the referrals have established relationships with the athletes that enable them to minimize the likelihood that the athletes will respond defensively and maximize the likelihood that the athletes will follow through on the referral.

For a variety of reasons, including lack of time, personal characteristics (e.g., tough-mindedness), possible loss of sport status, and public visibility, referral is an especially sensitive process. Consequently, it is important for those making referrals to be aware of the worries and anxieties that athletes being referred might experience. Such concerns can sometimes be alleviated by explaining in clear terms the reason for the referral and giving the athlete an idea of what working with the mental health professional will be like, thereby increasing the likelihood that the athlete will be able to save face and maintain dignity in a difficult, potentially embarrassing situation. Coaches and sports medicine practitioners can enhance the effectiveness of their referrals by developing referral networks in which they identify local specialists in clinical issues commonly encountered by athletes, become acquainted with the specialists and the way they generally work with clients, and, finally, provide athletes being referred with a description of what to expect from treatment.

Assessment

Once a referral has been made to a mental health practitioner and the athlete follows up on the referral, the first thing that is likely to happen is that the practitioner will interview the athlete about the nature of the presenting problem (e.g., history, duration, frequency, intensity). A recommendation for the athlete to complete one or more standardized psychological test—of the athlete's cognition, emotions, behavior, or some other relevant factor—may follow. The exact focus and methods of the practitioner's assessment of the athlete will depend primarily on the specifics of the athlete's presenting concern and the practitioner's theoretical orientation. The results of the assessment are typically used by the practitioner to diagnose the athlete's problem and formulate a treatment plan.

Diagnosis

In arriving at clinical diagnoses, mental health professionals compare information gleaned through assessment about athletes' cognitive, affective, behavioral, physiological, and social functioning with criteria for recognized categories of psychopathology set forth in diagnostic manuals such as the mental disorders section of International Statistical Classification of Diseases and Related Health Problems (ICD) and the Diagnostic and Statistical Manual of Mental Disorders (DSM). By itself, the receipt of a psychiatric diagnosis has no implications for the sport involvement of athletes, as many individuals are able to continue competing successfully despite their clinical conditions. Diagnoses enable practitioners to communicate with each other in a common language, help athletes to explain and understand the nature of their concerns, and provide practitioners with guidance on treatment options for the athletes in their care.

Treatment

Treatment of athletes with psychopathology varies widely as a function of the clinical conditions exhibited by the athletes and the particular practitioners to whom the athletes have been referred. In general, however, athletes are likely to receive at least one of several common forms of biological or psychological therapy. Treatment is generally conducted on an outpatient basis, but more severe types of psychopathology (e.g., those involving psychosis or dangerous behavior) may require inpatient treatment. Treatment is likely to continue until the focal clinical concern is resolved or stabilized, with follow-up treatment occurring as needed. Although extreme biological methods, such as electroconvulsive therapy or psychosurgery, are sometimes prescribed as treatments of last resort for certain intractable conditions, the most common type of biological therapy is psychotropic medication. Usually administered by a psychiatrist or other medical professional, pharmacological treatments are available for many mental disorders. Medication typically does not "cure" athletes of their psychopathology, but can lead to a reduction in symptoms and facilitate other forms of

treatment that can produce more lasting change. In addition to affecting the targeted clinical problem, medications often have side effects such as drowsiness, constipation, and dry mouth, all of which can interfere with sport performance. A special consideration for pharmacological treatment of athletes with psychopathology is the need for the prescribing professionals and the athletes alike to attend to and work around the list of banned and restricted substances for participants in the specific sports in which the athletes are involved.

For most forms of psychopathology in which a biological treatment is prescribed, it is typical also for some form of psychological treatment to be administered. The foci and methods vary considerably across psychotherapies. Among the most common, versatile, and effective forms of psychotherapy are behavior and cognitive therapies, which are often integrated in "cognitive–behavioral therapy" and are highly compatible with most performance enhancement interventions in sport psychology. Behavioral treatments involve the application of learning theory to help athletes shed maladaptive and/or acquire adaptive behaviors and emotional responses, whereas the emphasis in cognitive approaches is on identifying and modifying athletes' counterproductive patterns of thought in an attempt to produce desired emotional and behavioral outcomes.

Summary

As human beings, athletes are susceptible to psychopathology. Disorders involving anxiety, depression, eating, and psychoactive substances are among the more common clinical conditions experienced by athletes. Gender, age, and culture (including the culture of sport) are several of the factors that influence the occurrence of psychopathology in athletes. For athletes exhibiting signs of psychopathology, referral to a qualified mental health practitioner is warranted for subsequent assessment, diagnosis, and treatment. Attending to the clinical issues of athletes can help to maximize their well-being both on and off the field of play.

CASE STUDIES

CASE STUDY 1

Athlete

Christopher was a 17-year-old ice hockey player competing in the top non-professional league in his country. A tenacious defenseman, he was known for his fearless play and almost manic energy on the ice.

Reason for consultancy

In the course of conducting performance enhancement workshops for the squad, the sport psychology consultant noticed that Christopher blinked frequently in a pronounced manner and had an apparent tic in which he seemed to shrug his shoulders in an exaggerated way. The consultant had previously observed that Christopher made a lot of grunting noises while playing hockey, but at the time attributed the noises to Christopher's intense style of play. Although not clinically trained, the consultant had completed coursework in psychopathology and knew that Christopher seemed to fit the main diagnostic criteria for Tourette's disorder, a condition involving multiple motor and vocal tics. Consequently, the consultant discreetly scheduled an individual meeting with Christopher to discuss the matter further.

Background

Although initially hesitant to talk with the sport psychology consultant, Christopher seemed almost relieved when the sport psychology consultant expressed concern regarding his behavior. When asked about how long Christopher had been affected by his tics, Christopher indicated that he did not remember exactly when they began but that it was sometime after age 10 and that the severity had intensified over the years. He recalled having acquired the nickname "Wink" at age 14, adding that the nickname stuck with him when he changed teams. Christopher stated that although his tics seemed to get worse when he was "stressed out," he did not think that the tics impaired his sport performance. He speculated that his grunts on the ice may even help him by distracting or intimidating his opponents. He said that his main problem was that he had "compulsions" that he could not control. Christopher proceeded to describe touching rituals that he performed in the locker room prior to practices and games, and at home on a daily basis. Although he indicated that his teammates did not bother him about his rituals (noting that some of his teammates had even more unusual pre-performance routines than he!), he confessed that the rituals made him feel like he was "crazy."

Intervention

After learning the details of Christopher's situation, the sport psychology consultant suggested that there was a distinct possibility that Christopher might have a treatable neurological condition and that further evaluation was needed to be sure. Christopher reacted with a combination of relief and disbelief—relief that his situation could conceivably be explained and disbelief that there actually might be something that he could do

about it. Christopher willingly accepted a referral to a psychiatrist with whom the sport psychology consultant was acquainted and who had previous experience of treating elite athletes. Upon meeting with Christopher, the psychiatrist confirmed the diagnostic hypothesis of the sport psychology consultant and prescribed a low dose of an alpha-2 adrenergic agonist permitted for use by the World Anti-Doping Agency. The psychiatrist recommended that Christopher continue with the workshops that the sport psychology consultant was conducting and that he could make a conscious attempt to generalize the stress management skills he was learning in the sport context to his everyday life, enlisting the consultant to support Christopher's efforts in this regard.

After meeting with the psychiatrist, Christopher informed the sport psychology consultant that he wanted to disclose his condition to his coaches and teammates. The consultant discussed the pros and cons of such disclosure with Christopher and, satisfied that Christopher understood the ramifications of his intended course of action, facilitated a team meeting in which Christopher calmly educated the team about Tourette's disorder and his treatment. His coaches and teammates responded supportively, and one teammate asked "Dude, is this that disease where you shout out curse words and stuff?" Christopher replied that, yes, it was that disorder, but that he did not have that particular symptom and, unfortunately, could not cite the disorder as an excuse for using profane language. He informed the team that he was not offended by his nickname (although some people with Tourette's disorder would be), noting that he knew his teammates used the name without malice and that he himself had grown attached to it.

Outcome

Christopher tolerated the medication well and experienced a general reduction in symptoms, although he sometimes felt that the drug took away a portion of his "edge" on the ice, an observation not substantiated by external observers. His tics were not eliminated completely, however, and he occasionally found himself lapsing into his old rituals. Christopher was usually able to steer himself away from ruminating on his rituals by using the stress management techniques that he learned in the sport psychology workshops. The team, despite Christopher's proclamation to the contrary, used his old nickname only infrequently, and by the time he had advanced to the next level of competition, Christopher found that the nickname had been left behind.

CASE STUDY 2

Athlete

Chantal was a 23-year-old road cyclist of considerable talent. A member of an ethnic minority group in her country, she had risen from humble beginnings in an impoverished rural area to win a junior national championship in her specialty, the time trial.

Reason for consultancy

While completing a strenuous timed ride as a member of the national team at her country's high altitude training camp,

Chantal crashed on her bike under mysterious circumstances. Although she was not badly injured and sustained only superficial wounds, she was groggy when the support crew reached her and reported having no memory of the crash or the events that led up to it. Chantal displayed clear signs of dehydration, which she attributed to "a virus or something" that she had not divulged to her coach. The medical evaluation provided no evidence of brain injury, although testing revealed an elevated blood–alcohol content. A clinically trained sport psychology consultant assigned to the national cycling team was called in to provide support for Chantal.

Background
After emerging on the scene with her unexpected junior national title, Chantal had performed inconsistently, rarely putting together consecutive strong finishes in competition. The coach of the national team had selected Chantal for the high altitude training camp on the basis of her prodigious talent. At the camp, Chantal had mostly lagged behind her teammates in training, but occasionally showed flashes of the rider the coach believed she could be. She tended to isolate herself from her teammates, who, after Chantal's crash, informed the coach of Chantal's breakup of the relationship with her boyfriend back home, her withdrawal from team social activities, her occasional late-night angry outbursts, and her apparent consumption of large quantities of alcoholic beverages (based on the empty bottles they had found in her room when they went to bring some clothes to her in the hospital).

Intervention
While visiting Chantal in the hospital, the sport psychology consultant arranged to meet with Chantal 2 days after her release from the hospital. Chantal showed up for the session 20 min late and was quiet and somewhat lethargic but generally responsive during the initial interview. The consultant attempted to establish contact and build rapport with Chantal. While gathering basic information about Chantal's current situation, the consultant inquired about Chantal's relationships with her teammates. Chantal replied that although her teammates were friendly enough, she had not "connected" with them. She offered

that the women on the team were not as much fun as her friends back home. The consultant asked what Chantal meant by "fun." Chantal responded that she understood that cycling was important, but that her teammates never liked to "party" even when they did not have to awaken early in the morning to go on a ride. The consultant inquired about Chantal's use of alcohol, to which Chantal denied that she had a "problem with alcohol" and asserted somewhat defensively that she had been consuming no more alcohol than she had when she was performing at her best. Chantal acknowledged that some of her relatives had experienced alcohol-related health difficulties in the past, but dismissed these problems as "par for the course" for members of her ethnic group. At the conclusion of the session, Chantal agreed to meet again with the consultant several days later. Chantal missed the appointment and, in a follow-up telephone conversation, said that she would meet again with the consultant after the national holiday weekend (and team-approved absence from camp) slated to begin the next day.

Outcome
The sport psychology consultant, suspecting that Chantal was abusing alcohol, encountering difficulty adjusting to the training camp environment, and possibly experiencing a mood disorder, planned to discuss Chantal's drinking behavior and psychological state in greater detail at the next appointment. Unfortunately, Chantal never returned to the training camp. The coach informed the consultant that Chantal had packed up her belongings, left for the holiday, and had not returned. Telephone calls to Chantal's family confirmed that she had returned to her town of origin, but no direct contact was made with Chantal despite repeated attempts. The consultant was disappointed with the circumstances of Chantal's departure, but was informed by the sport governing body that athletes in other sports with backgrounds like Chantal's had met similar fates. Spurred on by what had happened with Chantal, the consultant developed an athlete support program to facilitate the adjustment of attendees from diverse cultural backgrounds at the country's national training centers.

Further reading

Brewer, B.W., Petrie, T.A. (2002) Psychopathology in sport and exercise. In J.L. Van Raalte & B.W. Brewer (eds.) *Exploring Sport and Exercise Psychology*, 2nd Edn, pp. 307–323. American Psychological Association, Washington, DC.

Gardner, F., Moore, Z. (2005) *Clinical Sport Psychology*. Human Kinetics, Champaign.

Solomon, G.S., Johnston, K.M., Lovell, M.R. (2006) *The Heads-Up on Sports Concussion*. Human Kinetics, Champaign.

Stainback, R.D. (1997) *Alcohol and Sport*. Human Kinetics, Champaign.

Thompson, R.A., Sherman, R.T. (1993) *Helping Athletes with Eating Disorders*. Human Kinetics, Champaign.

Chapter 10
Child and adolescent development and sport participation

Diane M. Wiese-Bjornstal, Nicole M. LaVoi and Jens Omli

Tucker Center for Research on Girls & Women in Sport, School of Kinesiology, University of Minnesota, Minneapolis, MN, USA

Psychological, social, and physical development processes project powerful influences on sport participation, defined broadly as engagement, learning, and performance in sport. Understanding these processes and the developmental trajectories of children and adolescents helps coaches work more effectively with the young athletes in their programs. Both maturational and environmental factors influence the progressive development of children and youth. Biological and experiential maturation factors need accommodation as part of effective sport skill instruction, and physical and socio-cultural environment influences can be advantageously structured to maximize the positive physical, mental, and social gains associated with participation in sport programs. Although the broad field of developmental psychology encompasses human growth and behavior change across the lifespan, the focus of this chapter is on discussing some of the developmental psychology issues affecting sport participants during childhood and adolescence, as these are formative years for the development of most sport skill proficiencies.

Developmental sport psychology is the term for the area of study focused on (a) exploring maturation and experience-related patterns of development in psychosocial factors affecting sport participation, (b) determining the role of sport participation experiences in developing psychological, social, and physical competencies, and (c) demonstrating how

Sport Psychology. 1st edition. Edited by Britton Brewer.
Published 2009 by Blackwell Publishing.
ISBN 978-1-4051-7363-6.

important social and task influences within the sport environment can be structured to enhance mental and physical development. The acquisition of sport skill expertise is both a product of development and a process for development, meaning that psychological development affects sport skill acquisition and that the sport skill acquisition process results in psychological changes. For example, psychological development affects sport learning and performance through maturation-related improvements in factors such as memory and perspective taking, and, participation in well-structured sport activities leads to improvements in specific psychological factors such as moral judgment and movement confidence. Effective coaches work with athletes and structure their programs in ways that advantage these developmental processes.

In the context of sport participation, important developmental considerations include the evidence-based beliefs that children are both quantitatively and qualitatively different from adults in maturation and experience and sport participation results in various developmental outcomes. The majority of the research upon which this chapter is based involves athletes from predominantly middle and upper-middle socioeconomic class populations in countries such as the United States, Canada, England, and Australia. In an attempt to mitigate cultural biases, an effort will be made to introduce principles of child and adolescent development that appear to transcend culture.

The purposes of this chapter are to (a) identify some of these quantitative and qualitative differences in cognitive, social, and psychomotor development, and explain how they influence the sport engagement, learning and performance of children and adolescents and (b) describe some examples of how important social influences can be used to maximize effective climates and instructional strategies that will accommodate and benefit the psychosocial and physical development of young athletes. This knowledge can be used by sport professionals in helping children and adolescents maximize their sport potentials to the extent they desire and are motivated to commit to their improvement and development.

Global models of sport participation

In the broadest sense, a macro-systemic developmental perspective viewed through the lens of elite international competitions such as the Olympic Games and current rosters of professional sport teams around the world provide a reminder that multiple developmental paths to sport participation and excellence exist. At least historically, the ways sport talent has been identified and developed in various parts of the world have been influenced by the ideology of countries in which the programs exist. Three models of sport talent development are described along the lines of cold war era geopolitical order.

The First World model of sport talent development, common in countries such as the United States and Australia, is characterized by high levels of participation across social classes at young ages, followed by continually decreasing participation levels as athletes become older and progress toward more elite levels of competition. In the First World model, youth sport is used to provide recreation and learning opportunities for many children and, for a few individuals, the opportunity to receive a university scholarship or professional contract. At each level of competition, the First World model involves a relatively high degree of organization and volunteerism by parents and other adults. Although some youth sport leaders do earn their incomes as officials, administrators, or coaches, a "parent as coach" model predominates at the younger age levels. It is worth noting that this chapter is based heavily on research conducted in

the context of the First World model of sport talent development.

Compared to the First World model, the Second World model of sport talent development is a more intentional way of developing elite athletes. The Second World model has been present in Russia and China, and the history of this model can be traced back at least to 1919 when V.I. Lenin established the first Institute for the Study of Sport and Physical Culture in St. Petersburg, Russia. It was here that some children were trained by a staff of professional coaches—many of whom were former competitive athletes who had gone on to receive graduate degrees in the exercise sciences—to compete in international competitions with the objective of demonstrating the strength of the Communist system. Due in part to the practice of identifying sport potential at early ages, fewer children enter into competitive sport training but consequently the rate at which athletes are eliminated from sport is lower than in the First World model in which peak participation occurs at around 13 years of age. The Second World model involves a high degree of organization and control by trained adults, many of whom earn their primary income through coaching and who coach within strongly autocratic systems of leadership.

The Third World model of sport talent development is the least proactive, but perhaps the most natural method of developing talented athletes, and is common in developing nations such as Uganda and the Dominican Republic. Compared to the First and Second World models, the Third World model involves far less organization and adult control, especially at the younger ages. Children participate in sport for the joy of participation and for something to do, but often, for boys at least, in the hopes of one day earning a living playing sport. They freely and imaginatively find ways to practice and play their sport in the available spaces and with often minimal or make-shift equipment but a high level of intrinsic motivation.

Though dramatic differences exist between each of these models in access, opportunity, structure, leadership, and training, the key point from a developmental perspective is that each model has and will continue to generate interest in sport participation among children and youth as well as produce world class athletes from a subset of these participants.

The success of these diverse models demonstrate that multiple and varied paths exist for the cultivation of sport engagement and the development of sport talent, and the path that is "best" is that which is a match between each unique child and the system in which he or she is raised. These models also serve as a reminder that although the development of sport talent is an important goal in and of itself, in the larger picture, the overall equity of sport opportunities provided and the engagement of a broad pool of youth in sport are equally important goals.

Cognitive development and sport participation

At the micro-systemic developmental level, the origin and the development of the sport-related capacities of athletes are affected by a complex interplay among genetic contributions, social climates, and physical environments. Cognitive development focuses on the maturity and growth of internal mental capabilities and functioning, such as thought processes, memory, motivation, and self-perceptions. These capabilities are essential to sport engagement and skill improvement, and understanding how they change with maturation and ecological exposure can help sport leaders more effectively structure their programs at an optimally matched level for the age and capacities of their athletes.

Cognitions

To best understand the psychological development of young athletes, it is helpful to look to two of the most influential research traditions in child development: (a) the intellectual stage theory of Jean Piaget and (b) the information-processing theories. Piaget suggested that development is driven by basic cognitive processes, including assimilation and equilibration. Assimilation is the process through which new information is adapted to existing ways of thinking. One form of assimilation—functional assimilation—is particularly relevant to youth sport, as functional assimilation occurs when children engage in behaviors for the sheer joy of mastering new skills. Children are naturally motivated to learn

and are rarely bored or "unmotivated" when offered the opportunity to learn new skills in a way that is challenging and interesting for them. Rather than using incentives, threats, or persuasion, coaches can keep children motivated by introducing challenging practice activities that facilitate learning.

Piaget suggested that learning occurs through equilibration, his term for the process through which children integrate disparate pieces of information from their world into an integrated whole. Equilibration can be summarized in three steps: First, the child is initially satisfied with existing ways of thinking (e.g., a young tennis player who believes that she should begin her service motion with her torso facing the target). Second, the child recognizes limitations in and becomes dissatisfied with existing ways of thinking (e.g., after watching more experienced athletes, the young tennis player realizes that a spin serve will be impossible unless she changes her service motion). Third, the child regains equilibration after replacing old ways of thinking with more complex ways of thinking (e.g., the young tennis player practices and masters the new service motion). Together, the processes of assimilation and equilibration allow children to progress through a typical series of developmental periods that span infancy to adolescence. Although development is not as stage-like as Piaget originally indicated, four developmental periods described by Piaget provide a helpful starting point to understand intellectual development in children. Because some organized youth sport programs start as early as 18 months of age, all four developmental periods are relevant to the present chapter.

Certain reflexes and other mental capacities are present prior to birth. During the first developmental period, the sensorimotor period (ages 0–2 years), the reflexes of children serve as a foundation upon which more complex mental capacities are built. During the sensorimotor period, children begin to imitate the motor behaviors of caregivers, discover that certain actions will bring about predictable consequences, experiment with different ways of manipulating objects, and begin to form mental representations of objects and events. Piaget noticed that toward the end of the sensorimotor period, children tend to reproduce behaviors with slight variations in order to observe different outcomes.

The ability to imitate behavior is fundamental to motor skill learning, as motor skills are often learned by watching coaches or other athletes demonstrate behaviors.

Representational ability, a key component of the second developmental period known as the preoperational period (2–7 years), is evidenced by "deferred imitation," in which children repeat a behavior modeled by another person hours after the behavior occurred. For children to learn from peer or coach demonstrations, they must have the ability to form a mental representation of the behavioral sequence. During the preoperational period, children are limited by egocentric thinking, such that they are not fully able to take the spatial perspective of others until the end of the preoperational period. Most young children are unable to imagine that someone standing in a different place on a football pitch would view an object, such as a goal, differently than they view the object. This limitation partially explains why young footballers may not notice that a teammate is open and is in a better position to score a goal.

During the third developmental period, the concrete operations period (ages 7–11 years), children develop the ability to represent transformation. In one of Piaget's most famous studies of the conservation of number, Piaget placed two rows of checkers next to each other (each with the same number of checkers) and asked children to indicate whether each row had "the same number or a different number." Piaget then asked the child to watch him spread out one of the rows of checkers. Once he had spread out one row of checkers, he again asked the child to report whether both rows had the same number of checkers or a different number. Most 5-year-olds reported that once one of the rows was spread out, the rows contained a different number of checkers. An ability to represent transformations is a necessary capacity for children to succeed in team sports such as basketball, which require players to watch and react as plays develop.

In the fourth developmental period, known as the formal operations period (11 years and older), children and adolescents develop the ability to entertain abstract concepts and imagine realities different from their own. The ability to consider concepts like meaning and truth also emerge during the formal operations period, allowing adolescents to think like adults. The advances that emerge during the formal operations period are a precondition for such sport tasks as learning a complex basketball offense or engaging in moral reasoning during adolescence and adulthood.

Memory

Although Piaget focused on intellectual advances that occur during childhood, information-processing theorists emphasize the development of memory systems. Unlike Piaget, most information-processing theorists contend that development is continuous rather than stage-like in nature. Information-processing theory focuses on "cognitive architecture," which is relatively enduring throughout development, as well as the efficiency of these structures in processing information. Compared to adults, information processing for children is limited by the amount of information that they can attend to simultaneously and the speed at which information can be processed. Different types of information are "stored" in different memory systems. Both adults and children are capable of storing vast amounts of sensory information from their environment for a short period of time. Sensory memory for both auditory and visual information increases with age such that 6-year-olds remember less sensory information than 9-year-olds or adults. Due to these limitations, it is especially important to be concise when speaking to young athletes.

Active thinking occurs in working memory, which is the system in which people manipulate information in order to comprehend language and develop strategies to solve problems. Working memory serves as a "processing area" where sensory information is combined with information from long-term memory to organize information in new ways. Working memory is limited in capacity—the amount of information that can be processed simultaneously and the length of time that information is held there. Older children can process more information in working memory than younger children, and can do so for longer periods of time. Limitations in their sensory and working memories help explain why most 3- to 5-year-old children appear to have "short attention spans." Although the sensory and working memories of young children are limited compared to adults, both adults and children have long-term memories that are virtually unlimited in capacity and duration. Long-term memory includes information about specific experiences (e.g., a child receiving her first trophy), rules (e.g., a ball that hits the white line on a tennis court is "in"), and procedures (e.g., the sequence of movements necessary to hit a tennis serve). Once children encode episodic, semantic, or procedural information in long-term memory, the memories often endure throughout the lifespan.

Motivation

Aside from the more general theories of child development, additional cognitive constructs, such as the personal motives of young athletes for sport participation, have been explored through the lens of other psychological and developmental theories. Competence motivation theory suggests that mastery behavior in activities such as sport is predicted by one's perceptions of ability and sense of control over performance situations. Youth sport participants typically have higher perceptions of competence and control than those who drop out. Achievement goal theory shows that behavior is often predicted by children's perceptions of their abilities and their goal perspectives, meaning their views on what it means to be "successful" in sport. Children and youth high in ego-orientation, an achievement focus that is other-oriented, often avoid challenges for fear of being viewed as incompetent by observers and only feel successful when they are superior to others. Task-oriented children and youth more strongly self-reference their perceptions of achievement, and thus typically better persist in their sport efforts because they are more focused on improving their own performances relative to their past abilities and performances than they are worried about how their success compares to others.

Children themselves give many specific reasons or motives for sport participation. Factors related to enjoyment are consistently listed by children and youth as among the most important reasons why they participate in sport. In addition to enjoyment or fun, they participate in sport to develop competencies, spend time with friends, improve fitness levels, experience challenges, gain new opportunities,

and bring honor to their families and nations. Conversely, it is not surprising that they quit sport when it is "no longer fun" or they are "no longer interested," or because of such factors as "lack of playing time," the "competitive emphasis in the program," or an "overemphasis on winning." Other children and youth discontinue participating in sport because they have "other things to do" such as homework and other extracurricular activities, perhaps a reflection on the dramatic increase in the time commitment expectations placed on many young athletes in recent years.

Youth sport attrition is often influenced by stress experienced while participating in youth sport. Possible sources of stress include self-perceptions, self-esteem, social evaluation, perceptions of goal-attainment, and parent and coach behavior at youth sport events. Among these social sources, angry parent behavior (e.g., yelling at officials) can be distressing for children, as the behavior can be a source of threat for young children and a source of embarrassment for older children. Likewise, the behavior of coaches can be a source of stress for children and has been found to have a significant effect on attrition. Coaches who create a climate centered on punishment, criticism, and favoritism have athletes who are more likely to drop out of sport than coaches who create a climate focused around contingent praise, encouragement, skill improvement, and equity.

In understanding long-term committed participation in sport, a distinction is often drawn between sport dropout, characterized by a withdrawal from sport participation due to a change in interest, and sport burnout, characterized by withdrawal from a sport due to chronic stress. Sport behavior is largely motivated by the desire to maximize the probability of positive experiences and minimize the probability of negative experiences. To maximize long-term interest and motivation, those responsible for structuring sport environments can do so in ways that keep children and youth interested in sport and that minimize the effects of chronic stress and negative experiences.

In the broadest participation sense, however, many children and youth throughout the world who would like to participate in sport never had the opportunity to do so because a variety of barriers stood in their way. These barriers include *sociocultural barriers* (e.g., sport participation is not deemed important in the society, perceptions that sport is not culturally appropriate for some youth [typically girls]), *access and opportunity barriers* (e.g., limitations in transportation, facilities, equipment, program offerings, or finances), *interpersonal barriers* (e.g., minimal caregiver support for sport engagement, parental belief that sport participation is less important than other activities), *psychological barriers* (e.g., limited confidence in one's physical abilities, little knowledge about sport, low perceived behavioral control over participation), and *time-based barriers* (e.g., too much homework, parental expectations for child to do chores or care for younger siblings). Policy makers and other influential adults could benefit the health and development of their children and youth through striving to reduce barriers to sport participation.

Self-perceptions

The cognitive perceptions that young athletes hold about their physical competencies affect their sport engagement. Younger children are generally more optimistic and older children are more realistic in evaluations of their competencies, with children's beliefs in their physical competencies declining over time. Children and youth rely on a variety of sources to gather information about their physical competencies. These sources change with age and as a function of certain psychological factors such as perceived competence and anxiety. During early childhood, children rely more predominantly on parent and spectator feedback and game outcome as information sources for knowing how good they are at physical activities. In later childhood and early adolescence, children demonstrate greater reliance on peer comparison and evaluation from peers and coaches. Later adolescence finds youth having greater dependence on self-referenced information about physical competence (e.g., effort exerted, goal achievement, skill improvement) and on a wider variety of information sources than at earlier ages.

Children's motivation for sport is affected by self-perceptions of their abilities in relation to the perceived difficulty of sport tasks. Early childhood athletes more typically use egocentric and self-referenced assessments of task difficulty, judging whether sport tasks are difficult or not based on whether they are hard for them personally. During middle childhood, children begin to adopt more objective levels or norm-referenced views of task difficulty, such that they recognize tasks that a few children can do are difficult and require high ability. In later childhood and early adolescence, children begin to believe that performance on tasks can be improved with effort, but they believe that effort is the cause of ability. From about early adolescence on, effort and ability are viewed as negatively related, meaning that if one has to work harder at something like a sport task, one must not have high ability. These beliefs affect athlete perceptions of their own competence and potential for future success, and thus affect their motivated behaviors in sport contexts.

In sum, cognitive development affects the sport participation of children and youth through many important mechanisms. Understanding thought processes, memory, motivation, and self-perceptions helps sport leaders match the demands of sport opportunities with the abilities of the young athletes.

Social development and sport participation

Social development looks at the nature and causes of how human social behavior develops as a function of both cognitive development and social experience. Trajectories in the development of interpersonal relationships, reactions to social climates, and effectiveness of group processes explain some of the differences in sport engagement, skill acquisition, and performance observed among children and youth.

Sports are inherently social contexts that intersect with other important social contexts such as family, education, community, culture, and economic systems. Research in child development demonstrates that children develop through shared activities such as sports. Children grow in and through connections with others, supporting the fundamental importance of warm, trusting, supportive, and close interpersonal sport relationships to overall well-being.

A scientific understanding of the development of social relationships helps practitioners understand how the social context of sport and the social agents within sports (e.g., parents, peers, siblings, coaches, fans, referees) interact with individual athlete differences (e.g., motives, goals, confidence) to influence cognitions, emotions, moral development, skill development, and sport performance.

Social development in early childhood

The genesis of many "sport careers" is in early childhood, often at around age five or six when children enter formal schooling. Children arrive in the social landscape of sport with developmental health assets and competencies derived from relational experiences during infancy, the toddler stage, and the preschool years. During these early times, parents and/or primary caregivers are important social agents that influence child development. Within the first year, infants have already learned the association between their distress, the caregiver's approach and soothing attention, and the infant's resultant comfort. Also within the first year, parental emotional cues are used by infants as a social reference that serves to help them clarify and interpret ambiguous events.

Attachment strength and security between children and their adult caregivers (usually their mothers) within the first year is believed to influence social, emotional, and personality development in subsequent years. Early relationships with available and responsive caregivers foster self-worth and self-efficacy, and aid in learning the skills, such as empathy and reciprocity, which are necessary for ongoing interactions with others. Attachment strength and adult responsiveness have significant effects on infant and early childhood social and emotional reactions, and provide the basis for a child's "internal working model." Internal working models of children generalize onto other relationships, such as extra-familial relationships (e.g., peers, coaches, intimate partners), and are strongly associated with children's abilities to form and maintain close relationships throughout their lives. Once children enter sport, relationships with key social agents, as further described, affect their subsequent development, sport participation efforts and accomplishments.

Parents and social development

Parents are typically the initial and most influential sport socialization agents for children. Mothers and fathers model their own sport participation and act as providers of sport experiences, supporters of sport participation, and interpreters of sport experience. Children consequently develop beliefs in their abilities, maintain certain expectations for their participation, and acquire sport-related value systems based largely on the influences of their parents. Parental encouragement, support, and praise have consistently been found to enhance children's perceptions of their abilities, enjoyment, interest, and involvement in sport. Conversely, unrealistically high parental expectations, excessive pressure, and frequent criticism have been linked to lesser enjoyment, interest, beliefs in abilities, intrinsic motivation, and greater perceived stress among youth athletes. Athlete perceptions of parental beliefs regarding effort, learning, enjoyment, and outcome provide situational cues about success and failure, which in turn influence athletes' achievement-related cognitions and subsequent sport behaviors.

Research has examined the effects of angry behaviors on children, such as inter-parental angry behaviors in the family context. These angry behaviors provoke distress and maladaptive responses among children, and are predictive of psychopathology and impairments in normal development. Therefore, if continuous sensitive care of adults over time is important for adaptive functioning, it likely follows that this is true outside of the private context of the family home, such as in the public context of sport participation. Parents at youth sport events often engage in undesirable behaviors such as yelling at the referee, yelling at athletes, and coaching from the sidelines. These behaviors are perceived by children and youth as distracting, annoying, and embarrassing. Negative parental sideline behaviors can produce stress, anxiety, and performance decrements in young athletes, and chronic exposure to these behaviors may result in undesirable consequences for them, such as psychological burnout or sport attrition.

Children's vulnerability to angry sideline behaviors may increase when their parents are also their coaches; thus these parent–coaches may be not only a source of angry parent behaviors but also the target of them. The rate of occurrence for this dual-role relationship is typically highest at the childhood and early adolescent levels—precisely when adult and particularly parental influence is most salient for children. Research indicates that children and youth report both positive and negative aspects of playing for a parent–coach. Regardless of the nature of the parent role in sport, parents remain the most important social influence in the development of their children. However, as children enter adolescence, the primary influence of the parent lessens, and peers and peer groups become increasingly important, as do social comparison and peer conformity.

Social development and peer relationships

Although parent influence on development is important, peer influence becomes increasingly influential through middle childhood and into adolescence. Establishing relationships with other children is a central task of early childhood, and given that sport is played within a context of friend and peer interactions, sport is a powerful context for social development. Sport participation provides opportunities for children to make friends, interact with diverse peers, play cooperatively, make comparisons that form competence beliefs, regulate emotions, and manage conflicts that may arise during the pursuit of collective or individual achievement goals. Research has demonstrated that friendship qualities in sport have both positive and negative dimensions, yet little is known about how perceptions of friendship qualities and peer relationship dimensions are linked to athletes' developmental outcomes.

Children with interpersonal attachments in which a sense of security is established and the core relationship strengths of stress resilience and emotional flexibility are formed are more likely to have positive and adaptive peer relationships. In early childhood, beginning at about age six, as cognitive and language skills expand, children's social skills grow in concert. As patterns of play move from functional non-social activity in infancy to cooperative games with rules in early childhood through adolescence, social skills are necessary for success, including sport participation success. Popular versus rejected children not only have different experiences with peers and social situations, but exhibit different patterns of development. Patterns of disruptiveness and antisocial behavior in early childhood predict aggressiveness and peer rejection and possibly early-onset delinquency later in their developmental trajectories.

Children who lack the social skills necessary to positively interact with peers, such as the abilities to take the perspective of others, sustain attention, regulate impulses, and manage conflict, are more likely than their self-regulated peers to be rejected by peers and develop early conduct problems. Unfortunately, children who lack social competence or self-regulation skills (e.g., children who have difficulty regulating emotions or behavior, or who do not feel accepted or a sense of belonging with peers) may be less likely to enter and stay in sport, or are more likely to be selected out of sport (e.g., cut from the team by coaches because of disruptive behavior). Subsequently, some children fail to have continuing access to the developmental benefits of sport because of their unsuccessful peer relationships.

Coach influences on social development

Children arrive at sport contexts through a developmental pathway largely governed in the early years by parent–child interactions and family climates. Once they enter sport, coaches have the opportunity to affect athlete development in two ways: (i) through the interdependent nature of coach–athlete relationships and (ii) through the climates they create. For children and adolescents who lack caring and secure relationships with adult caregivers at home, coach–athlete relationships may provide complementary or surrogate sources. Caring, supportive, and secure relationships with important adults such as coaches can convey protective influences against risk and lead to positive psychological outcomes such as emotional resiliency, personal empowerment, stronger self-worth, and capacity to deal with conflict.

Coaches can also facilitate development through meeting athletes' essential needs for belongingness, competence, and autonomy. Strategies employed by coaches to meet these athletes needs will vary across the developmental trajectories. For example, coaches cannot give the same amount of autonomy in decision-making for practice drills to 8-year-olds as they do to 18-year-olds and expect successful outcomes, due to variations in cognitive skills and experience. Similarly, fostering rapport and helping athletes feel cared about require age-matched strategies; to meet athletes' needs successfully throughout development requires technical and relational expertise on the part of coaches. The research of scholars exploring youth sport coach effectiveness demonstrates that coach expertise is trainable. For example, athletes who play for coaches trained to give positive reinforcement for performance and effort (care), and follow mistakes with encouragement (care) and technical instruction (competence) have been found to enjoy sport more, like their teammates better, and drop out less than those who play for coaches without such training. As athletes mature and reach higher levels of competition, they desire coaches who are both technically and relationally competent. This means that coaches must be knowledgeable about their sports and be able to teach and develop athlete skills, while simultaneously making athletes feel cared about and supported, and allowing them increasingly more input and self-governance as their autonomy matures.

Coaches can also influence athlete's development through the types of social-psychological climates they create. Research consistently reveals that athletes who perceive mastery (i.e., focus on learning, self-referenced standards of success) versus performance (i.e., focus on outperforming others, other-referenced standards of success) motivational climates as cultivated by the coach—regardless of age, gender, or competitive level—demonstrate adaptive achievement patterns and positive cognitive and emotional responses.

Moral development

Differences in moral understanding developed across these early years are likely related to the quality of later relational experiences with others. Moral understanding is fostered when parents and coaches help children to become aware of and learn normative standards of behavior in sport, and to interpret, label, and explain causes and consequences of emotion as well as social behaviors. The organization and content of parent–child and coach–athlete dialog is an important mechanism through which moral understanding develops. Through dialog parents and coaches build understanding, clarify causality and personal responsibility, and foster perspective taking, empathy, and the importance of cooperation with others. Perspective taking—perceiving the situation from the other's point of view—is an important social-cognitive skill, and good perspective takers are generally well-liked by their peers. During early childhood, children can begin to adopt the perspective of another person and recognize that others can do the same. By adolescence, the ability to step outside a two-person situation (e.g., knowing that the referee must hate it when people yell at him) is replaced by the ability to view self and others from a third-person perspective (e.g., knowing that Sam must feel embarrassed when his mom screams at the referee from the sidelines), and by early adulthood a societal perspective emerges (e.g., knowing that it is not right to scream at the referee because the referee is a human being who deserves everyone's respect). These stages also closely reflect stages of moral reasoning—the reasons individuals give to explain actions.

Moral development is also influenced by coach discipline strategies. Strategies that are coercive and power assertive, and those which heighten athlete anxiety and defensiveness, are less effective than strategies that reduce threat to athletes and use reasoning and justification for compliance. Ineffective strategies, for example, may include publicly humiliating, punishing, or embarrassing athletes for rule violations and simultaneously failing to explain the rationale behind the punishment to the athlete or the team (e.g., "We're all going to watch while Jake runs sprints in his underwear until he throws up"). If coaches can neither rationally explain neither "why" they are punishing individual athletes or the team nor how the punishment relates to core values, evidence would suggest those actions to be ineffective. Rather than relying primarily on imposing will and power on athletes, coaches should strive to appeal to the collective "good and right," justify decisions, and make transparent their reasoning and decision-making processes. Moral reasoning is more likely to develop when coaches ask athletes to reflect on how their actions affect everyone on the team (e.g., "What would happen if everyone disobeyed curfew and went out drinking the night before a game?" or "What does this say about our team that one of our members thought it was 'okay' to break curfew?"), rather than only appeal to individual responsibility (e.g., "It was your choice to disobey curfew."). In short, how coaches punish reflects and communicates whom and what they value.

Employing democratic decision-making is another relational process by which coaches can influence moral development. Coaches may be leery of adopting a "power-with" (i.e., shared) model of democratic leadership and may worry that children, not to mention adolescents, are incapable of being responsible for themselves, let alone for others. Coaches fear anarchy may be the result of their letting go of the reigns of discipline, but embracing power-with leadership does not involve the surrender of responsibility, but rather the ability to provide autonomy support and guidance to the members of their teams. This also does not mean burdening children with decisions and responsibilities that are inappropriate for their stages of development, but making athletes partners in their own sport experiences. Involvement in decision-making helps children to develop as autonomous persons, and autonomy has to do with making decisions about what is right and good for oneself and others.

Decisions are made and allowed, however, within the broader motivational climates created by coaches. Research demonstrates that athletes who perceive the sport climates to be ones in which coaches value performances and outcomes over the processes of learning and self-referenced mastery are more likely to demonstrate unsportsmanlike behaviors. The degree to which important people—parents, coaches, and peers—in the lives of athletes believe, endorse or engage in good or poor sport behavior, is predictive of the beliefs and actions of the athletes "on the field." Therefore, coaches who construct a "win at all costs" climate are more likely to have athletes that will, for example cheat to win and believe it is justifiable to do so.

In sum, social influences such as parents and coaches can use an understanding of social development to enhance the sport participation experiences of children and youth in two primary ways: (i) through the development of warm, caring, and supportive relationships with their athletes and (ii) by constructing and maintaining moral and mastery motivational climates. When these two dimensions are deliberately constructed by adult sport leaders working together with parents, a host of positive outcomes typically accrue for young athletes, including greater enjoyment, higher self-esteem, positive emotions, sustained and committed participation, more mature levels of sportsmanship, positive psychosocial and psychomotor development, and reduced competitive anxiety. In addition to fostering social development, both moral and motivational strategies simultaneously foster intrinsic motivation, the presence of which increases the likelihood that long-term commitment and optimal psychomotor development and performance will result, as further described.

Psychomotor development and sport participation

Learning sport skills is an educational process, and understanding the psychological aspects of effective teaching and learning helps coaches understand how to best encourage sport participation and develop motor and sport skill in their athletes. The acquisition and the performance of motor and sport skills in childhood and adolescence are critical to lifetime movement literacy, psychomotor confidence, and competitive success. Two important dimensions of psychomotor development include understanding: (i) how children develop motor skill and sport-specific abilities given maturational and experiential processes and (ii) effective educational strategies for maximizing this sport talent development. Sciences underlying these dimensions include motor learning (how motor skills are acquired and perfected), motor development (maturation and ecological processes underlying motor skill acquisition), motor control (control of motor skill by the neurological system), sport psychology (motivating athletes who want to participate in sport and to learn and improve motor skills), and educational psychology (employing effective ways of facilitating motor skill acquisition and knowing how to optimize motor skill learning through instructional strategies).

Psychomotor skill

Sport skills are a specialized subset of motor skills. At young ages, children benefit from a broad foundation of general motor skills, whereas with increasing age they naturally and typically begin to choose a few sport activities in which to develop more skill. Many elite athletes evidence a pattern of broad-based physical activity participation throughout their childhood years that lays a foundation for their later expertise, rather than intense and exclusive sport specialization at early ages. In general, it is advantageous to engage in this rudimentary form of cross-training early in life, when the goal is to develop an adaptable bandwidth of movement competencies that provide the groundwork for later motor specificity and specialization.

This pattern of broad participation in the early years, though, is somewhat dependent on the specific sport and the desired level of skill attainment. Studies from a variety of sports show that variability in athletes' physical maturation status has a strong influence on early sport success, providing an advantage in some sports, such as football and hockey, and something of a disadvantage in others, especially for girls participating in sports such as gymnastics or diving, which favor a pre-pubertal physique. However, the fact that success in sports such as gymnastics and figure skating requires intense early training and a career that peaks in puberty is a function not only of the demands of the sport and the physical and psychological capacities of athletes at certain ages, but also of the fact that the social influences of governing boards lead to them choosing to adopt rules and judging criteria that reward physical maneuvers that may force young athletes to excel early before their bodies mature, specialize in one sport at a young age, accept and play with injuries, and follow the dictates of authoritarian and sometimes abusive coaches and parents in the quest for elite status and achievement.

Sport talent

Coaches and other adults play a critical social role in influencing young athletes' efforts toward developing expertise in sport performance. In order to achieve elite levels of sport skill performance, some researchers have estimated that athletes must accumulate ten thousands hours of "deliberate practice"—described as effortful practice usually guided by a coach with the goal of facilitating performance improvements—over at least a 10-year period. This process is characterized by increasing amounts of practice time invested as athletes move up to higher levels of competition and age. Although intense commitment and preparation are necessary to achieve world class sport performance, researchers in this area also say that young athlete development programs must concurrently provide sufficient periods of mental and physical rest to allow for mental and physical recuperation, tissue regeneration, and avoidance of injury.

Intrinsic motivation for improvement also is inherent in the development of expert levels of sport skill. Retrospective evidence demonstrates that early in the careers of many elite athletes, they spent more time outside of organized practice sessions working on their individual motor skills than did their ultimately less elite counterparts. A composite of research on sport practice would lead to a rough estimate of approximately 4–6 practice hours per week outside of organized practices spent by these future elite young athletes on their individual motor skills from about 8 to 12-years of age. Additive to the physical practice effects, these unstructured child-centered times are driven by intrinsic motivation and behavioral choice, and they allow opportunity for the development of creative play-making and decision-making skills required in so many sport activities, but often stifled by a rigid focus on coach as decision maker in organized sport practices and competitions.

Scholars have argued that early sport talent identification cannot be achieved exclusively by traditional discrete or single-item assessments (such as coach-judged tryouts), but rather requires a complex and dynamic systems approach that embraces the role of developmental processes and variable paths to excellence in sport. Under this system, the emphasis is on sport leaders continuously assessing the changing learning potential of young sport participants rather than relying on highly time-isolated, genetically driven indicators of sport performance that are heavily influenced by physical maturity and individual differences in biological trajectories. Current systems for the early identification of sport talent are developmentally constrained by their emphases on short-term adult-governed assessments and expectancies, such as through holding sport team tryouts, cutting athletes from teams, and emphasizing coaching practices that invest more time with the "high talent" young athletes from the earliest of ages. The consequence is that many children and youth with great developmental sport potential are prematurely eliminated from organized sport, either directly through coach-related de-selection or indirectly through their own loss of confidence in their sport competencies following such de-selection and their subsequent limited expectancies for future success. Scholars from the United Kingdom and elsewhere have emphasized that youth sport talent identification strategies should focus on multiple dynamic assessments of physical, motor, and psychological dispositions, and their capacities to develop across transitions in individual athletes. The powerful social influences exerted by the evaluations of coaches during such sport talent identification processes should be focused on maximizing opportunity for development and improvement among a broad base of young athletes, for reasons related both to advantaging their personal growth and development and to their sport talent development.

Coach effectiveness

Expert coaches who get the most out of their young athletes employ a variety of educational and psychosocial strategies that make them effective. These strategies include those related to social psychology (e.g., creating effective and motivating learning climates that match the preferences of the athletes), cognitive psychology (e.g., understanding how much information to provide to learners at different levels of psychological development or what to expect of their attention spans and performance levels), and educational psychology (e.g., effective teaching of motor and sport skills).

One of the key instructional techniques used in sport skill acquisition is that of giving demonstrations, also referred to as observational learning or modeling. Effective sport skill demonstrations that involve both showing and telling young athletes how to perform sport skills correctly can greatly improve athletes' efforts, although the specifics of how and when to use these demonstrations are somewhat specific to the sport task and to the age of the athletes. From a biomechanical standpoint, there is typically a range or bandwidth of effective mechanical approaches to a specific sport skill contingent upon the anatomical, physical, and developmental profile of the individual athletes (e.g., their physical maturation, stature, and flexibility) and the constraints on the skill performances imposed by the sport rules (e.g., the requirement to keep the feet on the ground during a football throw-in). Demonstrations can serve the very useful function of conveying key motoric information about what to do quickly and effectively, and general recommendations for giving demonstrations include such considerations as repeating the demonstration more than once, giving the demonstration at actual speed before slowing down and then reconstructing to full speed, and using brief and descriptive verbal cues to cognitively connect the observer to the few most critical motor aspects of the performance. Again, depending on the sport, there may be some advantage conveyed by downplaying emphases on the outcomes for beginners and rather focusing more on the critical aspects of the form and timing of the movement (e.g., developing greater speed in a softball pitcher is advisable before an extensive emphasis on developing greater accuracy). Demonstrations are also typically more interesting to observers than merely listening to verbal instructions, and so convey a motivational advantage as well. In addition to their usefulness in showing athletes what specific sport skills look like (as many beginning young athletes may not have ever seen a specific skill performed before), demonstrations are helpful in showing athletes what particular drills look like so that they can quickly be organized to replicate the drill themselves. Demonstrations can also be used to develop perceptual–cognitive skills and game intelligence by directing athlete attention to demonstrations of opponent patterns of play or to view offensive or defensive sequences from the perspective of the performer. The key consideration seems to be that demonstrations should give the learners the idea of what to do and direct their attention to the most critical aspects of a performance. It is also important for demonstrations not to unduly constrain the performance of athletes to be required to perfectly match that of the demonstrator or model in order to allow for individual variability in maturity, development, and mechanics.

The ways in which physical activity leaders give feedback about motor performances once athletes begin their own practice efforts affect athlete psychological responses. Augmented feedback is the general term used to describe feedback provided by extrinsic sources such as coaches. Informational feedback provides skill-relevant information in response to physical attempts, and can be in the form of descriptive feedback, which "describes" what just happened, and/or prescriptive feedback, which "prescribes" how to fix errors or how to maintain good performances for the future. Evaluative feedback places judgments of approval or disappointment on the performances (such as praise, criticism, or ignoring). How athletes interpret these types of feedback and the consequences for their perceptions of competence and ability appear to be moderated by a variety of factors such as age and sport experience. Feedback affects athletes through their perceptions of physical ability, effort, and future expectations for success. Research has shown that coaches benefit athlete participation through their extensive use of positive, contingent, supportive, informational feedback combined with low punitive feedback. They detract from athlete participation with an overemphasis on ignoring (no feedback), negative feedback, and punitive feedback. Thus, as mentioned earlier, well-executed feedback is critical to establish task-focused and positive environments to generate longer term commitment to sport participation.

Expert coaches of children and youth seem particularly adept at knowing when and where to use the key behaviors of silence, praise, encouragement, and instruction in developing their young athletes. Quality (rather than quantity) instruction and feedback, punctuated by periods of silence and contingent praise, appear to be the characteristic of

effective coaches based on a composite of literature using observational assessments. From the perspective of the athletes, interviews with children and youth show that they are very clear and consistent about what they prefer their coaches to do and be. A good coach, according to young athletes, has the personal traits of being credible, nice, and fun; and behaviorally assumes competently the roles of manager, teacher, trainer, and performance enhancement specialist.

But even with the best of coaches and instructional strategies, not all sport participation can and should be adult structured, even for the maximization of sport talent. Children and youth gain much from the opportunity to practice and participate in sport activities without adult intrusion, or with minimal adult intrusion such as that provided by guided discovery and ecological approaches to coaching. As stated earlier, there are multiple models of sport participation and talent development, some of which have limited adult leadership until later in the athletes' development. The psychology literature demonstrates that there is variability of developmental windows of maturation and experience within which elite levels of sport skill can be achieved. Adults who establish rules and standards for sport development programs are encouraged to use that power in ways that recognize and benefit the physical, mental, and social development of children and youth.

Adversity and coping

Young athletes who are more resilient and are better prepared to handle adversity in sport engagement, learning, and performance will be advantaged in their development for and through sport. For example, excessive stress leads to physical and mental consequences such as fatigue, injury, decreased enjoyment, and emotional control problems. Learning to cope with adversity in sport is necessary to maintain and enjoy continued participation. Coping consists of those cognitive, emotional, and behavioral efforts used to manage difficult life situations. A variety of these difficult situations arise during sport participation, such as injury, abusive coaches, performance setbacks, and competitive losses. Three dimensions of coping with the stress and anxiety of sport situations have been identified: (i) problem-focused coping (trying to change the situation), (ii) emotion-focused coping (managing the emotions associated with the situation), and (iii) avoidance coping (removing oneself from the situation). Minimizing perceptions of excessive stress by providing a more positive and task-involved climate and developing coping and social resources among athletes are important mechanisms by which continued participation in sport can be achieved. In addition to the strategies described earlier for creating optimal psychosocial climates, individualized mental skills training programs as organized and implemented by sport psychologists are another effective way of preparing athletes to cope with difficult sport challenges. These programs typically include both cognitively and somatically based strategies for controlling stress and dealing with adversity, in addition to proactively developing mentally tough approaches to sport participation and competition. For example, psychological skills training programs often teach athletes to use mental skills such as imagery, goal setting, relaxation, self-talk, emotional control, and automaticity in effective ways for alleviating stress and enhancing performance. These self-regulatory psychological skills are essential to enjoyable and competent sport performance, just as they are for older athletes.

Life skills programs are another approach that has been used to help athletes develop broad bases of psychological and social skills necessary not only for coping with the challenges of sport participation but for broader life situations as well. Most of this chapter has focused on how child and adolescent development processes affect sport participation. This reciprocal path of influence—that is, that sport engagement, learning, and performance are not only achieved through the developmental readiness of athletes, but that they also develop athletes—is equally important. A positive youth development approach focuses on how sport participation can strengthen a variety of life assets for young people. In addition to the most obvious life skill assets of gaining motor competency and sport skill, sport participation can also be used to promote social, emotional, cognitive, behavioral, physical, and moral competence; foster resilience, self-efficacy, and identity; and develop connection and civic engagement in ways that extend far beyond the sport engagement.

Experiences and qualities central to positive youth development include building specific developmental health assets, all of which can be garnered through properly structured sport opportunities and climates. Developmental health assets or life skills typically include positive assets gained through the social climate and social institutions (e.g., supportive others, personal empowerment, behavioral boundaries, constructive use of time) and personal assets or skills generated through positive experiences (e.g., commitment to learning, positive values, being skilled in interpersonal and social interactions, feeling good about oneself). Having a greater quantity of developmental health assets relates to positive and successful youth development across a variety of contexts. Although not explicitly identified in most existing models of developmental health assets or life skills, unique groups of desirable benefits or assets attained through the context of sport participation should also include a more explicit focus on key physical assets, such as movement literacy, physical and mental health, physiological capacities, motor skills, and physical activity competencies. Beyond the sport performance benefits to having these assets, they also convey similar advantages to youth development across a broader variety of life situations. In sum, psychomotor development through effective instructional and educational practices is central to youth sport participation.

Summary

Figure 10.1 depicts a summary view of the aspects of development influencing sport participation among children and adolescents. Understanding athlete development as readiness for, process during, and outcome of sport participation, is the key to effective coaching and teaching of young athletes. This chapter described developmental psychology issues in a way that will help coaches use their knowledge of development to (a) structure effective progressions of mental and physical training and (b) hold realistic expectations of their athletes given their cognitive, social, and psychomotor developmental levels. By keeping these principles in mind, the sport talent of young athletes across the world can be developed to best advantage.

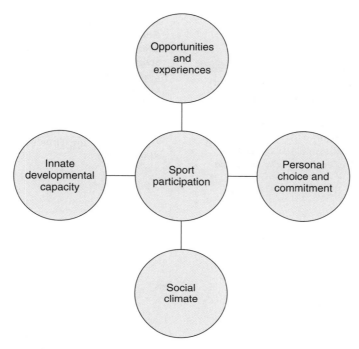

Figure 10.1. Developmental influences on child and adolescent sport participation

The following case illustrates how some of the principles in this chapter can be applied in sport settings for children and youth to achieve better physical and psychological outcomes.

Athletes
Beginning football players, about 5–7 years of age.

Background
Parents, coaches, and other adults working with young football players in a rural community recreation program meant well, but shouted loudly and created a somewhat heated context during Saturday morning football games as their children played competitive contests. A sport psychology professional was approached to offer recommendations for adapting the program to better match the developmental needs of the young athletes.

Professional assessment
In the opinion of the sport psychologist, the goals of recreational football programs at this early age group from a psychological perspective are to generate a love for the sport, offer opportunities to experience success, and instill a desire to keep playing the game without premature deselection. Socially, the goal is to minimize stress and anxiety for the young athletes who

are learning skills in a very public context. Psychomotorically, the goal is to have children maximize individual touches on the ball to develop football skill competence.

Intervention
For reasons related to psychological and social development, it was recommended by the sport psychology consultant that teams at this age should not have goal keepers, as this is a very stressful position associated with "winning" and "losing" in this public setting and is not well matched to athlete readiness for this specialized play. Another psychological advantage of no keepers is that it is exciting and very motivating to score goals, and without keepers more children would have a chance to score. For reasons related to psychomotor development, the consultant recommended that they play small-sided football, with fewer players per team and smaller play spaces thus allowing more frequent contact with the ball by all players and reflecting the fact that their kicking skills are just beginning to mature at this age.

Outcomes
After pilot testing the proposal for the first year, the local youth football association decided to continue the recommended practices for future years, as the children and families involved reported liking the changes and feeling that the desired objectives were achieved.

Further reading

Abbott, A., Collins, D. (2004) Eliminating the dichotomy between theory and practice in talent development and identification: considering the role of psychology. *Journal of Sport Sciences* **22**, 395–408.

Jowett, S., Lavallee, D. (2007) *Social Psychology in Sport*. Human Kinetics, Champaign.

Sroufe, L.A., Egeland, B., Carlson, E.A., Collins, W.A. (2005) *The Development of the Person: The Minnesota Study of Risk and Adaptation from Birth to Adulthood*. Guilford Press, New York.

Tucker Center for Research on Girls and Women in Sport (2007) *Developing Physically Active Girls: An Evidence-Based Multidisciplinary Approach*. University of Minnesota, Minneapolis, MN, viewed 20 December 2007, <http://www.tuckercenter.org/projects/tcrr/default.html\>.

Weiss, M.R. (2004) *Developmental Sport Psychology: A Lifespan Perspective*. Fitness Information Technology, Morgantown.

Chapter 11
Sport career termination

Albert J. Petitpas

Department of Psychology, Springfield College, Springfield, MA, USA

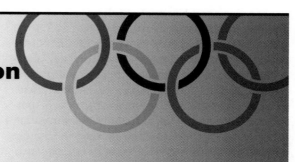

Introduction

William is facing a tough decision. Even though he is only 27 years old and coming off a bronze medal winning performance in the last Olympic Games, he does not know what to do. Should he spend another 4 years training for the 2008 Games, or "maybe it's time to grow up and finally get a real job" like all his university friends? He has to admit that it would be tough to imagine putting his body through another 4 years of countless hours of aches and pains. On the other hand, what in the world could ever replace the sheer joy of standing on the podium and receiving an Olympic medal?

Like many Olympians, William is at a crossroads in his sport career. Although he does not know yet what he will decide, he does know that someday in the not too distant future he will have to face the inevitable fact that his competitive sport career is coming to an end. The purpose of this chapter is to examine the sport career termination process. In particular, the following questions are addressed: (a) What are the causes of sport career termination? (b) What are some of the typical reactions that elite athletes experience when they leave competition? (c) How can athletes who are most likely to have difficulties with sport career termination be identified? (d) How can athletes prepare to cope with sport career termination?

Sport Psychology. 1st edition. Edited by Britton Brewer.
Published 2009 by Blackwell Publishing.
ISBN 978-1-4051-7363-6.

Causes of sport career termination and implications for coping

Although the longevity of a sport career varies by sport, most athletes face the inevitable decline of their abilities to compete both physically and mentally at a relatively young age. Ironically, elite athletes are often ending their sport career at about the same time most of their age-mates are just establishing themselves in their work careers. Although the deterioration of physical abilities would appear to be the most obvious cause for retirement from elite sport competition, there is general consensus among sport researchers that retirement is typically a result of multiple factors. The three most direct causes of sport career termination are deselection, injury, and free choice. The first two factors are not under the direct control of the athlete and typically result in an unplanned or involuntary termination. On the contrary, freely chosen retirement is often a more thoughtful and lengthy process in which athletes are better prepared to adapt to the transition out of elite sport. Often, there are differences in the experiences of athletes whose sport career termination was involuntary as opposed to freely chosen. These differences have proven to be quite useful both for predicting those athletes who may have the most difficulty in adjusting to the end of their sport career and for planning and implementing programs to prepare individuals for this transition.

The most frequent cause of involuntary disengagement from sport occurs during the team selection process. During each preseason or competitive trial, numerous athletes are "cut" from or fail to make teams. This deselection can cause emotional reactions ranging from denial and anger at the selection process to depression and despair. Unfortunately, those athletes who are most vulnerable to the selection process because of borderline or declining physical abilities are most apt to increase their training and become even more focused on their sport. One of the indirect consequences of placing primary or exclusive focus on sport is that educational or career planning gets pushed further into the background. As a result, the athletes who are most vulnerable to deselection are often the ones who are least prepared to cope with the end of their sport career.

Career-ending injuries are the second major cause of forced or involuntary termination from competitive sport. In many ways, a career-ending injury tends to be most difficult to manage and can lead to the most severe reactions. An acute career-ending injury is sudden, unexpected, and beyond a person's control—all factors that have been shown to lead to feelings of anxiety. The level of anxiety that is experienced relates to the amount of predictability and control that individuals perceive that they have over the situation. Considering this, it is easy to see how career-ending injuries can be so difficult to manage. In support of this belief, there is the consistent research finding that the former athletes who report the most life dissatisfaction after their sport career has ended are those who experienced career-ending injuries.

There are a number of other situational factors that can lead to sport career termination. Disqualification because of major National Governing Body (NGB) infractions, changes in coaching staffs, boycotts, financial problems, and family crises and commitments are just five of the reasons given by elite athletes for leaving their sport. These situational factors can be a direct cause (e.g., banned from competition because of a drug infraction) or an indirect cause, as in situations where these types of factors lead to deselection as a result of performance decrements.

The smoothest transition from athlete to nonathlete status typically occurs for those individuals who freely choose to retire from competition. Athletes who choose to end their sport careers usually do so because it fits into their own timetable. Many researchers refer to this type of disengagement from sport as an "on-time" transition. Typically, this type of transition occurs when athletes are at an appropriate age, have achieved their major sport goals, and have prepared for and planned what they will do after they retire from sport. Athletes who freely choose to retire add a degree of control and predictability to their transition experience that reduces some of the anxiety and uncertainty that could otherwise be expected in any major career transition.

In general, the process of sport career termination from elite competitive sport, whether freely chosen or forced, requires individuals to deal with many changes. How athletes react to these changes can vary in many ways.

Reactions to sport career termination

Although most individuals make a relatively smooth transition out of sport competition, the intensity of individuals' reactions to ending a career as an elite athlete can vary markedly. Many former elite athletes report that they miss many aspects of their sport career, specifically the competition, the camaraderie with teammates and coaches, the adulation of fans, and the total experience of participating in events such as the Olympic Games. Often, there is some sadness associated with the loss of sport and the realization that nothing will be able to duplicate the experiences inherent in being an elite athlete. Although only a very small percentage of athletes are likely to experience enough loss to manifest itself into clinical levels of depression, many others will second-guess their decision to retire or express some bitterness or sorrow if they believed that they were forced to leave sport before they had achieved all their sport goals.

One common reaction to the end of a sport career is confusion or questioning of one's self-identity. How do athletes define themselves if they are no longer in the role of "Olympic athlete," which can be a central source of personal and social identification? This is a question faced by many athletes as they transition out of elite competition. The further elite athletes move away from their sports, the more they may experience the need to develop a new identity or to learn to define themselves other than strictly in sport terms.

Many athletes find it necessary to make significant social adjustments when they leave elite competition. Frequently, other athletes, coaches, or sport-related individuals (e.g., administrators, medical professionals) serve as the primary social support network for elite athletes. Typically, a significant portion of this network will have difficulty in understanding why a given athlete has chosen to retire. Adding geographic changes and separation from teammates, it is not hard to understand that athletes may also experience some loneliness or boredom as they readjust to life without elite competition.

Elite athletes are also used to fairly regimented schedules. They typically know what to expect from year to year, and much of their lives revolve around a set routine of practice, competitions, and other related commitments. As a result, many retiring athletes are not prepared to cope with the ambiguity of an uncertain future and may lose confidence in their abilities to meet the demands of establishing themselves in a non-sport career. This loss of confidence is often accompanied by fear or anxiety emanating from the belief that they are years behind their age-mates in work experience.

Another common reaction to sport career termination is a feeling of emptiness or lack of purpose. For many years, elite athletes are typically focused on reaching a specific goal. Whether the goal is to win a medal or to simply make the Olympic squad, these athletes have a clear sense of direction and purpose that brings meaning to their lives. Once retired, athletes may feel empty inside and question if all the time, effort, and struggles were really worth it. Some athletes, particularly those who feel they were forced to retire, can drift from activity to activity in the hopes of finding a new sense of direction. Others may become bitter at the sport system and disown their entire sport experience or find it too painful to even follow their sport on television or through the media. Still others will attempt to hold onto their sport by becoming involved in coaching, broadcasting, or sport administration. Nonetheless, those athletes who are able to place their sport participation in perspective appear to be in the best position to harness the positive energy from their sport experiences, which helps ease the transition into their next career.

Predicting athletes who are most likely to have difficulty with sport career termination

Sport career termination is a transition, and as with any transition, athletes who retire are forced to cope with change and make adjustments in how they view themselves and the world. Most athletes cope with these changes relatively easily, but a small number struggle and experience enough distress that they may become clinically depressed, abuse substances, develop eating disorders, or incur other emotional or physical problems. Although predicting those athletes who are likely to have the most difficulty in adjusting to sport retirement is not a foolproof science, there are several factors that have been shown to lead to higher levels of vulnerability to distress during sport career termination.

Although several researchers have described various stages in the career progression of elite athletes, all of these models contain a period of specialization in which athletes narrow their focus on sport participation. This devotion and commitment to excel in sport allows athletes to perfect their techniques and enhance their performance. However, if the strength and exclusivity of this specialization becomes too great, athletes can fail to engage in other activities that have been shown by research to be critical in developing a cogent sense of personal identity.

As individuals move into late adolescence and early adulthood, their primary developmental task is to explore different occupational, ideological, and life roles. During this exploratory period, individuals learn valuable life skills, build self-esteem, and gain a better sense of their values, needs, interests, and skills. Exploratory behavior not only provides individuals with the skills, confidence, and self-knowledge that are necessary to make commitments to a personal identity, but also exposes them to experiences that increase their abilities to cope effectively with life transitions and other stressors. Unfortunately, the rigors, time commitments, and focus necessary to excel in sport may prevent many elite athletes from exploring non-sport roles.

Athletes who have the greatest gap between their level of aspiration and level of ability may be particularly vulnerable when faced with the threat of the loss of sport. These individuals often believe that they cannot afford to take any time or attention away from their sport. Therefore, instead of planning for their future or exploring other roles or activities, they become more strongly and exclusively focused on their sport. In other words, they essentially put all of their hopes and dreams in their athletic identity. They typically ignore objective feedback about their chances of achieving their goals, withdraw from their athletic social support network, and devote even more time and effort into practicing their sport skills. As a result, the occurrence of a career-ending injury or deselection can be particularly traumatic.

Another factor related to adjustment to sport career termination is the amount and quality of life/work planning that athletes engage in prior to leaving sport. Athletes who fail to plan for the future often believe that they are years behind their age-mates in establishing themselves in the workplace. They typically lack the self-awareness that accrues from exploratory behavior and have a limited sense of their values, non-sport interests, and skills. With no clear plan or sense of direction, these athletes can lose confidence and fall into a state of apathy. They often report feeling a sense of emptiness and have difficulty in taking the initial steps necessary to engage in career exploration.

Although the strength and exclusivity of the athletic identity, the amount of exploratory behavior, and the extent of future planning are all indicators of athletes' development, the quality and availability of a person's social support network and the resources available in the individual's environment are also important factors in adjusting to sport career transitions. As stated earlier, the major segment of an elite athlete's social support network is often comprised of people who are involved in elite sport. These sources of support can be quite beneficial during the sport career, but they may not be as helpful during the process leading up to retirement or after the end of the sport career.

Research has shown that the more similarities in make-up and interest among members of a support network, the more limited the range of assistance that can be offered. The term "density" is commonly used to describe the level of similarity among the support group members. Individuals within a high density support group tend to know each other and hold similar values and beliefs about what is needed in specific situations. The density of elite level athletes' social support networks is often quite high, as the networks tend to be composed primarily or exclusively of athletes, coaches, and sport administrators. These individuals may be more invested in keeping athletes involved with sport, rather than in facilitating their transition into retirement. In addition, coaches and teammates are typically excellent sources of informational support and challenge, but they are often limited in their abilities to provide emotional support. As a result, those athletes, without a broad and diverse support system, may not have the types of support necessary to assist in managing the emotions or in making the difficult decisions that are frequently involved in the process of ending a career as an elite athlete.

A final factor that can influence the impact and consequences of ending a sport career is the resources available to the athlete within the setting in which the transition occurs. Sport environments with appropriate sports medicine or athlete assistance services can provide the support and resources necessary to ease the transition out of competitive sport. These services are particularly vital in situations where the individual athlete lacks the internal resources or social support required to cope effectively with sport career termination.

Assisting athletes in preparing for or coping with sport career termination

Even though it may be possible to identify those athletes who are most susceptible to distress when coping with the termination of their sport careers, it can be quite difficult to get the most at-risk athletes to participate in prevention programs. These individuals are often reluctant to devote any extra time or energy to activities that are not directly related to improving their sport performance. Therefore, when planning support programs to facilitate a smooth transition out of competitive sport, NGBs and other sport organizations should consider several types of services.

The Life Development Intervention (LDI) model provides a helpful format for planning support programs for athletes. The LDI perspective views transitions as a process rather than as a discrete event. For example, sport career terminations begin when athletes first think about ending their sport career, continue during the retirement process, and extend through the aftermath of adjusting to life without competitive sport. As such, a comprehensive support program should have different components that are available before, during, and after a transitional event. Programs that assist athletes in preparing for a future event are called enhancement strategies. Those programs that take place during the event in an effort to buffer the impact of the transition are called support strategies and those that take place after the event to help athletes cope with the aftermath of the transition are called counseling strategies.

The cornerstone of any comprehensive transition program is enhancement. For elite athletes, enhancement services assist them in preparing for sport career termination by helping them identify the skills they have acquired through sport, showing them how these skills can be used in different life areas, and by teaching new skills that can enhance their abilities to cope with all the changes that can occur as a result of disengagement from sport. By preparing for their eventual retirement from competitive sport, athletes are better able to anticipate some of the changes that they might experience and gain confidence in their ability to cope with these changes.

A number of Olympic Committees throughout the world, including those in Australia, Canada, the United Kingdom, and the United States, have created programs to assist athletes in preparing for their inevitable retirement from sport. Although each of these programs is structured differently, they all share some common goals. In general, these programs aim to assist elite athletes by (a) providing a supportive environment in which they can share their concerns; (b) helping them to identify their values, needs, interests, and skills; (c) assisting them with life/career planning; (d) building their confidence in their abilities to make a successful transition into a new career; and (e) establishing an accessible support group of other athletes, coaches, or sport administrators. In particular, athletes who participate in Olympic-sponsored career development programs report that they benefit from activities in which they identify their transferable skills and learn how to transfer these skills into non-sport careers. It appears that when athletes believe that they have skills that are valued in the workplace, they gain confidence in their abilities and experience less anxiety when confronting their retirement from elite sport.

Unfortunately, it is not easy to get athletes to participate in life skills enhancement programs. There appears to be a pervasive fear among many coaches and athletes that any activity that is not directly related to improving sport performance may become a distraction and cause athletes to lose focus on their sport goals. This fear has not been substantiated by research. In fact, a study of Australian Olympic athletes showed that those who participated in a comprehensive life skills education program displayed more stable and consistent performance than their athlete peers who did not participate. Ironically, this research suggests that life skills development programs might actually provide immediate performance benefits to elite athletes.

Another benefit of enhancement programs is that through the self-assessment activities that are part of the life/work planning process, athletes often develop a more well-rounded view of themselves and begin to see themselves as more than exclusively athletes. Athletes who learn to explore and balance various life roles are typically more self-aware and are therefore in the best position to make informed decisions about their transition out of elite sport. Athletes who adopt an exclusive identity as an athlete are more apt to avoid enhancement programs and put off their sport career termination as long as possible. When this is the case, support programs should be made available to help these athletes cope while they are in the midst of their sport termination process.

A substantial number of athletes, particularly those who have not participated in any enhancement programs, experience strong emotions while they are disengaging from elite competition. Unfortunately, during the transition out of sport, many athletes report that very few people understand what they are experiencing. They often feel alone, sad, and anxious about their futures, but are hesitant to disclose their feelings to people who have not shared their sport experiences. Hence, it is important for NGBs to make support services available for those athletes who are in the midst of the sport career termination process. These athletes typically need to address how they are feeling in a forum where they feel that others understand what they are going through. This need can be attended to by organizing a group of athletes who are in the process of retiring from sport and inviting several former elite athletes who have already gone through the retirement process to meet with the group. The purpose of the group is to create a safe forum for self-disclosure by having several of the retired athletes share their transition experiences with the group. Although simply sharing emotions may not resolve any of the issues involved in the transition, it can be a necessary first step because some athletes can become emotionally paralyzed by the strong feelings that leaving sport can evoke.

A related issue is what has been referred to as the "Olympic self-image." Elite athletes who have been revered by fans and placed on pedestals can have a difficult time imagining themselves in anything but exciting and high visibility careers. These athletes typically fail to acknowledge all the time and hard work it took to progress up to elite levels of competition. The difficulties with this situation can be compounded when athletes also develop a sense of entitlement. If they have been overprotected and overindulged because of their sport skills, then they may not be willing to engage in career and life planning because they assume that the sport system will simply take care of them. In either case, they may refuse to start at the bottom level of a new career progression and experience anger and disappointment at what they believe is a sport system that has abandoned them.

Support and career exploration services provided by Olympic organizations can help buffer some of the negative feelings or self-image problems that can develop during sport career termination. Planning programs for normative transitional periods, such as immediately after Olympic trials and Games, can provide athletes with the support and information that can facilitate a smooth adjustment period. It is also important to monitor and follow-up with the participants of these support programs to ensure that they continue to work toward their new goals and have the required support available if they encounter any major roadblocks.

As described earlier, a small number of athletes experience enough distress over their sport career termination that they develop problems such as substance abuse, eating disorders, depression, or other clinical problems. Therefore, Olympic organizations or sport governing bodies should develop a referral network of professionals who can address these types of issues. Ideally, these professionals are not only specialists in dealing with individuals with the specific issue, but also have sufficient knowledge of the sport experience to understand how factors such as the strength and exclusivity of the athletic identity can affect functioning.

As shown in Figure 11.1, a comprehensive support service to assist athletes who are experiencing sport career termination should include components that (a) help athletes anticipate and prepare for their retirement; (b) provide an appropriate support network for athletes during the transition; and (c) establish a referral network of professionals who can assist athletes with specific problems that can arise in the aftermath of the transition. Clearly, enhancement strategies that help athletes prepare for the transition are the best means of facilitating a smooth sport career termination. Therefore, Olympic governing bodies that build these services into the normative experiences of their athletes are likely to have the most far reaching impact.

Conclusions

The purpose of this chapter was to examine the process of sport career termination. In general, adjustment to ending a sport career is influenced by a large number of factors. Chief among these

- *Enhancement*: Activities that can be done before sport career termination
  - Acquire life skills
  - Identify transferable skills
  - Conduct self-assessment to identify values, needs, interests, and skills
  - Begin life/work planning process

- *Support*: Activities that take place during the sport career termination process
  - Create a diverse social support network
  - Organize support groups of athletes who are coping with sport career termination and several former athletes who have already made the transition out of sport

- *Counseling*: Services that are available to athletes who need assistance with coping with the aftermath of sport career termination
  - Develop network of referral sources for issues such as substance abuse, eating disorders, and other forms of psychological distress
  - Maintain contact with retired athletes to keep them connected with sport support systems

Figure 11.1. A framework for planning interventions to assist with sport career termination

factors is the amount of planning and preparation athletes engage in prior to retirement, the degree to which they explore other roles and broaden their self-identity, the availability and quality of a social support network, and whether the decision to retire was voluntary or forced. Olympic governing bodies and other sport organizations that promote life skills education for athletes from the beginning of their sport careers greatly enhance the probability that their athletes will have a relatively smooth sport career termination. Athletes who fail to prepare for the end of their sport career and who are forced to retire are often in need of support services to help them manage all the changes that take place during the transition out of sport. In addition, a small percentage of athletes may require specialized counseling services to cope with the aftermath of a difficult termination process.

CASE STUDY

The athlete

Chris is a 24-year-old skier who had participated in the previous Olympic. Although he had been projected to be a potential medalist in the next Games, he was struggling to regain his form and had begun to get feedback that several of his teammates had already surpassed him. Even though the next Olympics were still 18 months away, Chris could feel that the pressure was increasing. To make matters worse, it seemed that the harder he pushed in practice, the poorer he performed. Chris could not bear the thought that he might not make the Olympic squad this time. Although skiing had always been the central focus of his life, Chris was becoming even more obsessive in his training, and spending more and more time working out and studying his technique. Eventually, the stress and extra physical pounding took its toll on Chris' body and he developed several nagging injuries that only seemed to exacerbate his declining performances. His frustration was rising and began to manifest itself in several angry exchanges with one of his coaches. Chris'

behavior was becoming incorrigible and teammates and coaches alike found it difficult to be around him.

Reason for consultancy

Eventually, one of Chris' coaches recommended him to see the team sport psychologist. Chris refused. He isolated himself from his teammates as much as he could and spent what little free time he had talking with a previous coach from his hometown. The previous coach had always taken a lot of pride in Chris' accomplishments and seemed to live out many of his own Olympic dreams vicariously through Chris. As a result, he was more than willing to offer Chris whatever advice he could.

Inevitably, the months passed and Chris did not qualify for the Olympic squad. He was devastated. He had devoted his life to becoming an Olympic medalist and he had nothing to show for it. He blamed his coaches and the NGB officials for playing favorites and not supporting him when he needed assistance. He was bitter and lost, and did not know what he was going to do next. He questioned whether his body could stand up to the rigors of four more years of intense training. On the other hand, skiing was all he knew.

After several months, Chris contacted one of the assistant coaches and asked about his status on the team. The coach listened to Chris' concerns and recommended that he speak with the sport psychologist because of all the things that had gone on the year before. Although Chris was reluctant to seek help, he also believed that he would jeopardize his chances of making the team even further if he ignored the coach's advice.

Professional assessment

Although Chris was somewhat defensive and hesitant to disclose his true feelings, he faithfully attended weekly meetings and gradually built a trusting relationship with the sport psychologist. Over the weeks, it became clear that Chris had such a strong and exclusive athletic identity that he had placed enormous amounts of pressure on himself to win a medal. He had alienated himself from his teammates and coaches, and relied almost exclusively on a previous coach who was more invested in getting Chris to the Olympics than in helping him deal with his current situation. As a result, Chris was desperate to fix his own problem, but ended up hurting himself by pushing too hard physically, withdrawing from his teammates and other sources of social support, and refusing to seek out professional assistance.

Intervention

After Chris was able to work through a lot of his anger, frustration, and sadness, he was referred to a life/work planning forum that was sponsored by a former professional athlete. During the forum, Chris learned how to conduct a self-assessment that not only allowed him to identify his values, needs, interests, and skills, but also encouraged him to define himself as more than simply an athlete. Chris also explored several career options and spent some of his free time as a management intern at a regional sporting goods company. During these experiences, Chris was able to identify and gain confidence in his ability to use his sport skills in the workplace. As a result of his hard work, Chris was allowed to continue to participate with the ski team during this period. He balanced his practices and workouts with his business internship responsibilities, and believed that each experience added to his emerging self-awareness.

Outcome

Chris made the next Olympic squad as an alternate and felt quite satisfied with what he was able to accomplish in and out of sport. He had made the decision that he would retire from sport competition after this Olympic event no matter what the outcome of the selection process was. Although he still missed the excitement of the sport, he was able to make the transition into his new management career relatively easy. Chris now serves as a resource person for other Olympic athletes who are dealing with sport career transitions.

Further reading

Danish, S., Petitpas, A., Hale, B. (1993) Life development interventions for athletes: life skills through sports. *The Counseling Psychologist* **21**, 352–385.

Chapter 12
Sport psychology in practice

Mark B. Andersen

School of Human Movement, Recreation, and Performance and the Center for Ageing, Rehabilitation, Exercise, and Sport, Victoria University, Melbourne, Australia

Introduction

Delivering sport psychology services, in the real world of athletes and coaches in individual and team sports, is a species of practice that, at times, is both similar to and at variance with other traditional forms of psychological consultation. Sport psychologists often work outside of formal offices or clinical and counseling settings. For example, a psychologist for an Olympic team may attend practices, sit in on team meetings, travel and stay at the hotel with the team, eat at the team dining tables with the athletes and coaches, and deliver services on the field in the middle of practices. The boundaries of the "where" of practice are often considerably looser than the traditional psychological services.

The "what," or the *content*, of service may also vary considerably in comparison to the more traditional forms of counseling. For example, the early model of sport psychology service delivery focussed primarily on interventions for performance enhancement, and that model is probably the one most prominent in many athletes' and coaches' views of what a sport psychologist does. So, an athlete or coach may initially seek out services for performance enhancement (e.g., positive self-talk, imagery, relaxation, goal setting), but that type of service may be just the entry point for athletes to start talking about other life concerns. As trust builds between the athlete and

Sport Psychology. 1st edition. Edited by Britton Brewer.
Published 2009 by Blackwell Publishing.
ISBN 978-1-4051-7363-6.

sport psychologist, the other issues may emerge that pull the service along new and decidedly non-sport paths. For example, a sport psychologist and a basketball player may spend months on performance enhancement work. They get to know each other better, begin to feel comfortable with their working relationship, and then (because trust has developed sufficiently) suddenly one day the athlete says "Hey, Doc, I really don't want to do imagery today. What I really need to talk to you about is my love life. It sucks." And then a story tumbles out about isolation, feeling awkward in the presence of potential romantic partners, low self-esteem regarding attractiveness, bumbling efforts at getting close to persons the athlete finds attractive, and repeated failures at intimacy. The service compass may then swing 90 or 180 degrees from sport to a whole other realm of the athlete's life. One hopes that the sport psychologist is capable of working with the athlete on intimate relationship issues (many are; many aren't). If the sport psychologist's service repertoire is only the cognitive–behavioral interventions of performance enhancement, then a referral to another expert is in order. If the sport psychologist is equipped to work on romantic issues, then the relationship changes, and probably becomes more intimate and personal than it was before the athlete revealed what was really bothering him or her.

The wonderful thing about sport psychology service is that it often provides a relatively non-stigmatizing path to work with a psychologist. Seeing a psychologist for sport-related issues (e.g., strengthening one's mental game), in many sport environments, is seen as a part of good training.

Seeing a psychologist for mental disorders still has a stigmatizing flavor. Past research, however, has shown that athletes do not look down on other athletes who see sport psychologists for sport-related concerns. Many sport psychologists tell stories about how athletes first come to them for performance enhancement, but then, as in the above mentioned example, after a month or two or three, the *real*, or more central issues emerge. One well-known sport psychologist has called this phenomenon of service change "the issue behind the issue."

Just as the physical and content boundaries of practice are varied, so too are the types of service delivered. This chapter will cover the various types of professionals and their training, the different clients they work with, the models they use in service, the personal qualities coaches and athletes want in their practitioners, and the foundations of successful practice.

Who are the professionals and where do we find them?

The answer to the first part of that question is there are many, and they come from diverse backgrounds. As for finding a sport psychology professional, word of mouth is one of the most common routes, but there are also professional associations that can be helpful in locating consultants. The international organization *Association for Applied Sport Psychology* certifies practitioners of sport psychology services. A list, with contact details, of their certified consultants can be found on their website: www.aaasponline.org. The *United States Olympic Committee* has a registry of sport psychologists. More information on their registry can be found at: http://www.usoc.org/teamusanet/TeamUSAnet_46377.cfm. The *British Olympic Association* and the *British Association of Sport and Exercise Science* also have registries of consultants.

People in psychology or psychology-related fields in sport settings are many and varied. They range from performance enhancement specialists to clinical psychologists, career counselors, and player welfare officers. Descriptions of some of the professionals who may provide psychological services to athletes, coaches, and teams are presented in the following section.

Service from a sport science perspective

The *Directory of Graduate Programs in Applied Sport Psychology* (Sachs et al., 2007) lists 100+ programs worldwide, and over 90% of them are housed in sport science (e.g., exercise science, human movement, kinesiology, physical education) departments. Sport psychology service from a sport science perspective has, in general, primarily a performance focus. Just as applied exercise physiologists try to determine which sort of physical training will produce the best results for athletes, sport science-oriented psychologists explore and deliver different types of mental training aimed at improving performance. Most of the practitioners trained through sport science programs are not licensed (chartered, registered) psychologists and do not call themselves "psychologists" (a legal and professional title protected in many countries).

With the majority of practitioners of sport psychology coming from a sport science perspective, the likelihood of encountering a professional with this background is high. Many practitioners with sport science training will state up front that they work in the area of mental training for performance enhancement, and that working with other inter- and intrapersonal issues (e.g., relationship problems, psychopathology) are not part of their services. If athletes and coaches are primarily interested in mental skills for improving performance, then there is an abundance of people with sport science training who would be available. The majority of consultants listed on the registries mentioned earlier have sport science backgrounds.

Service from counseling and clinical psychology perspectives

Counseling and clinical sport psychologists have usually received their training in psychology departments, or in some cases in education departments (e.g., counselor education degrees). The distinction between counseling psychology and clinical psychology is blurry at best. As a gross overgeneralization, counseling psychologists work with usually normally functioning individuals who are experiencing psychological difficulties in the areas of stress, adjustment, relationships, and other issues, but are not experiencing serious psychopathology. Clinical psychologists deal more with people who have diagnosable mental disorders. Nevertheless, the range of practice and the types of clients served by these practitioners, in reality, overlap extensively.

Clinical and counseling sport psychologists, in general, take a much broader perspective than a focus on performance. If athletes want to understand themselves, their motivations, their maladaptive patterns of behavior, and where sport fits and does not fit well in their lives, then a counseling specialist would be a more optimal choice than a performance enhancement psychologist. If the athlete's concerns move into the realm of psychopathology such as depression, eating disorders, distress due to personality disorders, and so forth, then a clinical psychologist would probably be the best practitioner to contact.

Others in the field

Life coaches

In the past two decades, the service profession of life coaching has grown internationally. There are now many different life coaching professional associations who certify practitioners (e.g., *Life Coaching Association of Australia*, *Association of Coaching* [United Kingdom], *US Life Coaching Association*). The main focus of life coaching is to help people plan and develop goals and to enable them to change behaviors in order to reach those goals. Certified life coaches are well-trained in one of the central interventions most sport psychologists use: goal setting. The legitimate life coaching literature and promotional materials specifically state that life coaching is about planning and reaching specific goals and *not* about clinical issues. Life coaches are trained in a circumscribed area of service, and do not (or should not) attempt to handle concerns outside the area of goal setting and behavior changes necessary to help their clients meet their goals.

One possible reason for the growth and popularity of life coaching is that the service does not

contain words such as *psychology* or *psychotherapy*. There is still a stigma attached to seeing a psychologist (something is mentally wrong with the person), but seeing a "coach" sounds both sporty and healthy, sort of like working with a "personal trainer" (see Section "Introduction" for a similar example of non-stigmatizing service). Coaches and athletes who have specific targets for training and performance may wish to use the services of a life coach to help them reach their goals. Life coaching, however, is not a holistic approach to athlete's care, but rather a service designed for specific aims. In many cases, a life coach may be all that athletes want or need to help them in their sport endeavors. As in all cases of hiring professionals, athletes and coaches need to check the credentials of the practitioners they are considering to employ. If a life coach is not affiliated with a national association, or has not received training from a certified life coaching institution, then his or her services are suspect.

Motivational speakers

There is no doubt that many motivational speakers can be, in a word, motivating. Before big games or major competitions, many coaches employ motivational speakers to give rousing talks to "fire up" the athletes for the upcoming challenges. The actual effect of such an intervention is unknown, and no research has been conducted to test the effectiveness of motivational speakers. Anecdotal evidence suggests that many athletes enjoy listening to someone who speaks positively about their abilities, but the jury is still out on whether motivational speakers have any direct or indirect influence on performance. The "jury" will probably be out for a long time because testing effectiveness of a usually one-off intervention is nearly an impossible task.

Many sport psychologists, in their careers, can report times when they have received calls from coaches and managers of teams they do not know, asking them to come down and "fire up" their athletes before a major competition. There are possible benefits and dangers in accepting such assignments. One danger is introducing something new to athletes just before the important events. Instructing athletes to change something (e.g., start using positive affirmations) or use new cue words in the upcoming competition introduces a new and unstable material to their competition rituals. Those new behaviors or thoughts may actually interfere with what they have solidly in their systems and lead to disruptions. On the positive side, and if the athletes do well later, the sport psychologist may be seen as valuable and someone who can contribute. On the negative side, if the athletes don't perform to the expectations, the latest event to get them motivated (i.e., the sport psychologist) may be on the receiving end of blame. Many sport psychologists have been on the receiving end of such requests for motivational talks, and they may be hard to resist, especially for sport psychology practitioners who are in the early stages of their careers. Saying "yes" to such requests is tempting because giving a motivational talk may be seen as an avenue to further contact with the team and future employment. In such talks with athletes and coaches, however, it is probably best not to introduce new material or approaches to competition, but rather to have the athletes focus on what they do well and remind them of all they have accomplished.

One of the reasons coaches often want to "pull out all the stops" and bring in a motivational speaker or other people to inspire the team is an attempt to cover all the bases, but an underlying motivation may be anxiety about the upcoming event and doubts about the team's preparation. The motivational speaker, in part, then becomes an anxiolytic (anxiety decreasing) intervenor, so the coaches, in the end, can say "I did everything I could." If the team does well, then the sport psychologist may get some credit (and future paying work). If the team does not do well then the sport psychologist may get some blame (e.g., for getting the team over-aroused). If the sport psychologist already has an ongoing relationship with the team and is well known to the players, then a precompetition "pep talk" probably does not carry near the risks of bringing in someone from "outside" the team environment.

Charlatans

A sport psychologist was working as a full-time practitioner for an American university intercollegiate sport department (600+ athletes in various sports), and he would get a call about once a month from someone who wanted to "help" him work with the athletes. Many of these people had little or no formal training in psychology or sport science, but indicated that they believed they had something of benefit to offer athletes and coaches. One gentleman offered, in all sincerity (he believed), to help adjust the "auras" of athletes because when athletes take off in planes to fly to participate in competitions, the acceleration misaligns their auras, and they would not be able to perform well until their auras were readjusted. The psychologist could just imagine how an athlete or coach would respond to such a service. The psychologist also amusingly wondered why the deceleration of landing the plane would not pop the auras back into place. The aura adjuster's offer was politely declined.

The above mentioned example is an obvious one, but many charlatans are much more subtle. Sport, and especially sport at the Olympic and professional levels, is a glamorous place that can attract people who wish to bask in reflected glory, or take some of the glory of sport success for themselves. These people are the ones coaches and athletes need to be wary of; they can do untold damage to athletes and teams. If any person comes unsolicited to a coach or sport administrator offering psychological services, then yellow, if not red, flags should start to wave. They may be legitimate practitioners seeking employment, but a thorough background check on training, university degrees, credentials, and references from past sport organizations about their services should be conducted. A major problem with the professional practice of sport psychology is that there are many charlatans out there who leave trails of alienation behind them and sour coaches and athletes on the potential benefits of the services that legitimate practitioners can provide. It is not uncommon to hear coaches say "We had a sport psychologist, and he was a total fruitcake. We'll never do that again."

The business end of service

Some sport psychologists have full-time positions with professional teams or with state and national sport organizations (e.g., United States Olympic Committee, Australian Institute of Sport). Many sport psychologists have academic positions and do consulting work in addition to their university duties. Most non-academic sport psychologists, however, work part-time for teams and individual athletes in a variety of settings and have private consulting practices.

Many coaches and athletes who would like to have the services of a sport psychologist do not have a lot of money. Some sport psychologists, especially those who are in the early stages of their careers, may offer services at substantially reduced rates. Another avenue for inexpensive or reduced-fee services is for coaches and athletes to contact academic institutions where future sport psychologists are being trained. The students in such institutions usually need to have field experience and may be available to work with teams pro bono. The *Directory of Graduate Programs in Applied Sport Psychology,* mentioned at the beginning of this chapter, is one of the best sources for finding such training institutions.

The ethics and professional practice codes of many countries' psychological associations recommend to members that at least a small part of practice for professionals should be delivered at low fees or pro bono, so even established sport psychologists may be available at reduced fees. Many of the ethical codes of practice in psychology discuss the problems associated with "bartering" for services (e.g., consultation "paid for" by season tickets or sport equipment). Usually, the recommendations are not to engage in barter, but that exceptions can be made (e.g., psychologists working in small communities or low-income rural settings). In those cases where teams are poorly funded, those exceptions to barter would possibly apply for sport psychology practitioners.

Sport psychology services, like most professional activities, usually involve a negotiation process between the deliverer and the client(s). That process may result in a formal contract with specified hours, types of service, and fee structures. In other cases, the parties involved may settle on a "retainer" fee for the whole season that would include, in one package, all sorts of services (e.g., observation time at competitions, consultations, one-on-one athlete

contacts, team seminars). Setting out the plan for fees for services right at the start is probably the best way to proceed from an ethical and professional practice point of view.

A final issue about business would be for the receiver of service to inquire about professional insurance. Most sport psychology practitioners who are registered (licensed, chartered) psychologists carry indemnity or malpractice insurance. It is unknown how many practitioners who are not registered psychologists have these sorts of professional protection. This issue of professional practice is probably not covered in many negotiations in the field, but, as in most cases in hiring professionals (e.g., plumbers, electricians), such considerations should be taken into account. *Caveat emptor* applies in sport psychology as it does in so many other areas where professional services and fees are negotiated.

Who are the clients and where are the boundaries?

At first glance, the question of who the clients are seems to have an obvious answer: the athletes. When examined more closely, sport psychology services may have several other stakeholders attached. For example, a parent may bring an athlete to a sport psychologist, but then also informally seek out the psychologist's advice on matters concerning the athlete. The official service is for the athlete, but the unofficial service is for helping the parent to cope with raising a superstar.

The loose physical boundaries of service mentioned earlier have their counterparts in the determination of who the client is. For example, a coach, at first, wants a sport psychologist to work with the athletes, but then later seeks out the psychologist, rather informally, for feedback on his or her coaching style. One problem in this loose delivery environment is that sport psychologists can slip into serving others without any formal recognition of what is happening. When sport psychologists feel that they are slipping into different service roles with other members of sport organizations or with parents, then instead of continuing to slip, it is wise to stop for a moment and discuss and renegotiate roles to help make boundaries and service clear to all parties. For example, a psychologist is working only with athletes on a team, and then about a month or two after service began, the coach approaches the practitioner and asks: "How do you think I handled that half-time talk?" Here is the time to stop and shift the conversation to clarifying the roles. The psychologist might say, "Coach, I think there was some really good stuff in your talk, and there were a couple of things I had questions about, but before we go into that, I need to get some clarification. I have been working only with your athletes up until now. With your question about half-time, I was wondering if now you would like me to work with you and have discussions and feedback on your coaching style. If that is what you want, then that sort shifts our relationship, and we will need to broaden the focus on what I observe and take mental notes on so I can pay more attention and thought to you. Let's discuss my role or roles on the team so that everyone is on the same page. How does that sound?" Boundaries and scope of service can easily become blurred in the loose environments of sport. Monitoring those boundaries, becoming aware of when the focus is not clear, and reclarifying the shifting qualities and types of delivery are all ongoing tasks of sport psychologists in service to athletes, coaches, parents, and sports administrators.

Athletes

Athletes are the most obvious people for whom sport psychologists may supply service. Athletes may, at first, present performance issues for the sport psychologists to "fix." They may come to the sport psychologist with preconceptions that their problems are something that just need some "tweaking" along the lines of a minor adjustment in a sport technique. They may come through a referral by the coach and be compliant or resistant. They may come self-referred, looking for someone to talk to who does not have any special agenda (e.g., winning a medal). They

may come to vent about frustrations with the team or coach.

Understanding the pathway through which the athlete arrived in the sport psychologist's office will give signposts about how to proceed. For example, if the athlete is coach-referred and resistant to being there, then continued service and building rapport may be difficult. Direct questions, such as "Do you really want to be here?" can be disarming. Assuring athletes that their attendance at such sessions is completely up to them, and that they do not have to talk about anything if they do not want to, can help the athletes feel more at ease and less defensive. In this situation the sport psychologist may say, "Well, the coach wants you to spend some time here, but I don't tell the coach anything about our sessions that you don't want him/her to hear. So why don't we use the hour in some way? Maybe you could tell me something about how you got started in sport. I'd be interested in getting to know about another member of the team." That sort of communication tells the athlete that the psychologist is not following the coach's agenda, and is there only for the athlete. Such a friendly and conversational approach may even lead to the athlete wanting to come back and talk some more.

There is probably a public misperception that athletes are relatively well-adjusted, high functioning, mentally healthy, and generally happy people. How could they not be? If they had "mental problems," then they could not perform like they do. The public often idealizes (and idolizes) athletes, especially those who are successful and in the media. The public "persona" of the high functioning athlete is worrisome. It can trap athletes in a cage of not seeking help because they don't want to tarnish that image, so many athletes struggle with personal difficulties alone and in silence. Athletes, however, are not these "superhuman" people. They have all the fears, joys, anxieties, loves, hates, hopes, sadnesses, and psychological issues that the rest of us have. In the best of all possible sport psychology service worlds, practitioners should be equipped to help more than the persona of the athlete and see the athlete as a whole person with both impressive strengths and accomplishments and human frailties. The readers of this chapter might want to read the autobiography of Greg Louganis or the biography of Patria Thomas. Those works are probably two of the most fully "human" accounts of the lives of athletes.

Coaches

The above mentioned example of a coach seeking a sport psychologist for consultation on coaching practices is only one form of service. In some systems of service (e.g., former Soviet bloc countries), the coach is the primary client with the sport psychologist supplying information about athletes (e.g., personality, coaching style preference, competitive anxiety, other psychological assessment data) to the coach so that she/he can help the athlete to reach his/her best. The sport psychologist in such a system is acting in a sport science role, just as a biomechanist or as a exercise physiologist would do as part of the support team. Such a system of service, however, raises questions of confidentiality and informed consent. Can athletes "freely" consent to having psychological information about them released to coaches? If athletes believe their positions on teams, or team selection may be determined, in part, by psychologists' reports, then a couple of things may happen. They may consent to please the coach and in response to team pressure (i.e., "coerced" consent, not "free" consent). They may also attempt to "fake good" on any psychological assessment tasks, rendering the assessments invalid. This form of sport psychology service to the coach is not the one that many current practitioners would embrace.

Some coaches have (an unfounded) faith in psychological assessment and what the results of psychological tests can predict in terms of athletes' performance or development. Many sport psychologists have been requested to test athletes for a variety of purposes (e.g., team selection, prediction of which athletes will develop well). Unfortunately, psychological assessment tools really don't have the power to do what some coaches think they can do. Coaches' misperceptions about psychological assessment may actually come from sport psychologists themselves. Some practitioners have produced their own psychometric tools and have marketed them to the coaches as ways to measure who will be the future superstars. The truth of the matter is that there are no psychological assessment tools that can reliably predict who will be successful, who will develop fast, or who will become a team leader. Some sport psychologists may sincerely believe that they have powerful tools to assess athletes, and some just fit into the above-mentioned category of "charlatan." The best advice for a coach, when approached by a psychologist claiming to have powerful assessment tools, is to "walk the other way."

Sometimes coaches seek out sport psychologists, not for their athletes, but rather for their own personal and professional reasons. Coaches, like all people, have their own psychosocial issues (e.g., relationship problems, anger control difficulties, depressed mood, job anxieties) and may seek out sport psychologists for counseling in areas other than their roles as coaches.

Whole teams

Often, especially in the early days of service, a sport psychologist may be employed primarily as a deliverer of psychoeducational sessions for the whole teams. Usually at the coach's or administration's request, the psychologist meets with the whole team to discuss mental skills for performance enhancement, such as relaxation, imagery, goal setting, and self-talk. One of the primary, but often unstated, goals of such psychoeducational presentations is that some of the athletes on the team may become interested and approach the sport psychologist for further one-on-one service. Many sport psychologists will deliver "lectures" on psychological skills to the team. This approach is probably suboptimal. A better strategy is to conduct the session in a way as interactive as possible. For example, if the topic were about relaxation, the sport psychologist might try to engage the group by asking for stories about when they were really playing well and up to their potential, followed by stories when they were nervous, tense, and their performance was below what they expected. Inevitably, stories will emerge about anxiety and "playing tight" that the sport psychologist can use to illustrate points about the benefits of learning how to stay relaxed and loose. Using athlete's stories to conduct psychoeducational sessions serves many purposes. Educational activities in which the "students" are active participants are almost always more effective than when they are passive recipients of information. Telling stories and having them appreciated and used in this process also helps to build rapport and leaves many athletes with the impression that the sport psychologist is interested in them personally and is one who cares for them.

Psychoeducational group presentations are ways of gaining entry to a team. Delivering them in an interactive, seminar format may increase the likelihood of further work with the team and the individuals.

Sport organizations

Sport psychologists, especially those with organizational psychology backgrounds, may be employed by National Governing Bodies (NGBs) to help with organizational and "team" communication issues. The sport psychologist may observe the interactions of different subgroups (e.g., coach–athlete interactions, head and assistant coaches' communications, management and coaching staff encounters), interview key stakeholders, and make recommendations for organizational changes. In such a case, the sport psychologist is brought in as a consulting expert in much the same way as organizational psychologists consult with businesses.

Parents

Parents usually want the best for their children, but they often have their own agendas that may come in conflict with the overarching agendas of the psychologists. For example, a parent may bring a child to a sport psychologist to "fix" the child's motivation to continue in sport. The parent may also be the one paying the bill. How does one handle the parent's desires, yet keep the focus on the health and welfare of the athlete. Following is an example of how psychologists might speak about their service with a parent and an athlete:

> When I work with athletes, my main agenda is the health and happiness of the person.

Sometimes that involves working primarily on mental skills like focus and motivation for performance enhancement. Sometimes the work is about improving communication with coaches or teammates. In all cases, the focus of what we work on, or talk about, is determined by the athlete. Many athletes I've met with have improved their performance, but some athletes I've worked with have not improved, and some have even decided that they would like to pursue other interests, scale back, or even leave their sports. There is no guarantee about the direction that our meetings will take because our sessions are directed by the needs and best interests of the athlete (from Van Raalte & Andersen, 2007).

Parents also want to know what is happening with their children and will often ask questions that sport psychologists cannot, without athlete permission, answer. Explaining confidentiality to parents is a delicate process. A sport psychologist might say:

> I always encourage the athletes I work with to discuss what we are doing with their parents and coaches, but I also tell them that if there is some stuff they don't want to tell their parents and coaches, then what they have to say stays only in the room with me and them. Some athletes may have some interpersonal or relationship concerns with the coach that they are not ready to talk to the coach about. Discussing these sorts of issues in a confidential setting helps build trust and lets the athletes know that I am not there for anyone except for them. Confidentiality is an ethical cornerstone of psychological service, and I am bound by my profession to honor privacy. Does that make sense to you?

In some local, regional and state sport organizations, parents of athletes also sit on governing boards. The dual roles of parent and sport administrator can make for interesting political maneuvering. Sport psychologists who work with athletes who have parents on the sport governing body can find themselves in professionally precarious positions.

The instruments of service

Sport psychologists have two major tools that they use in service. The first tool comes from the training, education, theoretical foundation, and models of practice they learned. For many sport psychologists, these tools stem from cognitive–behavioral theory (CBT) and practice. They guide sport psychologists in what to look for and how to address the issues the athletes present. Using a CBT model, practitioners listen for adaptive and maladaptive patterns of thinking (the cognitive part) along with exploring the contingencies of reinforcement and punishment (what is pleasing and what is displeasing about sport involvement) that maintain behaviors that are helpful (the behavioral part) and those that are not helpful. Whether sport psychologists use a CBT model, or any other model for service, it is the system they follow that helps practitioners to formulate athlete's concerns and guides the interventions to be implemented.

The second instrument of service is the sport psychologist him or herself. In the sport sciences, there is generally more emphasis on learning about the model-for-service instrument. In clinical and counseling psychology there is also an emphasis on learning models of practice, with an added focus on the personality and psychosocial history of the practitioner. In their training as psychologists, many students spend a great deal of time examining their own personalities, their patterns of behavior, their interpersonal skills and relationships in order to gain some understanding of themselves. The Socratic admonition to "know thyself" is a central feature in the process of becoming a psychologist.

The dangers in not examining the personality and psychosocial history of the sport psychologist are many. Without an understanding of personal motivations for becoming a sport psychologist, one's own unresolved issues around one's own sport career, the adaptive and maladaptive ways in which one interacts with others, and one's own emotional and interpersonal needs then the sport psychologist may inadvertently and unconsciously interact with an athlete in ways that meet the psychologist's needs more than the athlete's. Unfortunately, there are too many examples of sport psychologists using athletes, by proxy, to make up for their own perceived failings in their past sport careers.

Research has shown that coaches and athletes want sport psychologists who are knowledgeable about both sport and psychological interventions, who show genuine care for those they serve, who are flexible, and who do not have personal agendas (e.g., sharing sport glory). The descriptions of the "preferred" sport psychologist that athletes and coaches reported in research look, unsurprisingly, like the qualities that most people want in a psychologist. Many years ago, Carl Rogers, the founder of client-centered therapy, described the ideal psychologist as: having unconditional positive regard for clients, being truly empathic, being genuine, possessing authenticity, being nonjudgmental, and having a caring for, and appreciation of, human frailty. That description is an ideal to strive toward for all sport psychologists regardless of their education and training backgrounds.

The foundation of service: The working relationship

A central question in sport psychology service delivery for athletes, coaches, and psychologists is, "Can we work together?" In other words, "Are we a match when it comes to forming a working alliance?" The answer to that question is not a simple "yes" or "no," and then we proceed with the service or withdraw. That question probably has to be visited and revisited several times over the course of service, but the working relationship, or alliance, lies at the center of service.

In the related fields of counseling and psychotherapy, research has shown that the type of therapy used (e.g., cognitive-behavioral, family systems, interpersonal therapy) is not as important, in terms of outcome, as is the quality of the relationships between the practitioners and the clients. The one variable that seems to be the most important is how well the professional and the receiver of services get along with each other. For example, if the coach has "forced" the athlete to visit the sport psychologist, and the athlete is uncomfortable with, or even wary of, the psychologist, then the client may be unwilling to disclose any concerns and just go through the motions of seeing the practitioner to comply with the coach's wishes. In this case, much progress will not be made because there is really no working relationship. There is only suspicion and compliance. If, however, the athlete is willing and eager to engage in sport psychology work, likes the practitioner, feels safe, and forms a positive and mutually respectful relationship, then progress is likely to occur.

Trust, confidence, care, genuineness, and mutual positive regard are some of the central features of a salubrious working alliance. These qualities of the relationship may develop quickly, or they may evolve over several months. When two people come together to work on helping one person function better, there may need to be considerable time, along with ups and downs in the relationship, before a solid working alliance develops.

In a one-on-one psychological working relationship there are two experts involved. The sport psychologist is the expert in performance enhancement, counseling, or psychotherapy (or even all three areas). The athletes are the experts on their own worlds, perceptions, behaviors, and emotions along with probably greater expertise than the sport psychologist in the demands of the sports involved. There is, however, a power differential in that the sport psychologist is in the "helping" position and is acting in the role of a professional. That power differential may be abused, as in the case where the sport psychologist uses athletes for personal gain (e.g., reflected-glory, taking credit for athletes' accomplishments, using the athletes to work out personal past disappointments in the sport psychologist's own sport history, colluding with athletes in their conflicts with their coaches), resulting in professional and, most likely, damaging *misalliances*. The power differential can become less lopsided through acknowledgment of the athletes' expertise in both sport and their personal

worldviews. Sport psychologists can also help balance the power issues by asking the athlete to become the sport psychologist's "teacher" about the subtleties and nuances of the sport, the physical and psychological demands they face, and the tactics of competition. Such an approach also helps solidify that central feature of service, the working alliance.

Final thoughts on service

Sport psychology service is complex and multilayered. It has to be humans are messy, and what seem like simple and straightforward "performance" issues are more likely convoluted with possible deep roots extending beyond sport and competition. Those roots may be lodged in the soil of self-esteem, body image, contingent parental love, and feelings of unworthiness. These roots, however, do not necessarily have to be exposed. Just because there are problems elsewhere in an athlete's life, that does not mean they have to be addressed. As illustrated in this chapter, there are many types of services for many types of people involved in sport. The cardinal rule in any service is to "follow the client." The athletes and coaches (or whoever the clients are) will eventually take the sport psychologist to where they need to go. That journey may be a short and simple one, such as helping an athlete and coach to communicate better with each other. The journey may be a dark and stormy passage through the personal hell of early childhood trauma and repeated psychological and physical abuse.

The main issue for sport psychologists is to have a keen appreciation and deep understanding of which adventures they are equipped to undertake with their clients, and for which journeys they lack the gear and need to refer to another professional guide. Also, the needs of the athlete–clients stand far above the needs of the sport psychologist, and to paraphrase one of the field's modern founders, Bruce Ogilvie, in addressing sport psychologists and their work, "the extent to which you can lose your ego in service will influence how helpful you are to the athletes in your care."

CASE STUDY

The athlete

A 5000-m runner, April, came to see a sport psychologist on the recommendation of her coach. April knew the sport psychologist, Jenny, because she had presented some talks to the whole team on the topics of relaxation, imagery, and self-talk. April also thought it was a good idea to see the sport psychologist because she recognized that she had some performance difficulties. April was 19 years old and had been competing in distance running since she was 12. April's main concern was performance in competitions. Her coach had told the sport psychologist that April could pull out great runs in practice, but in competition, usually during the last two or three laps, she would start to fade and lose contact with the front pack of runners. April's stories about competition matched well with what the coach had reported.

The sport psychology consultant

Jenny had been practicing in the field of sport psychology for 14 years. She had received a master's degree in counseling and a Ph.D. in sport psychology from a sport science department. Jenny usually followed a cognitive–behavioral approach to performance enhancement, but also conducted a thorough interview about other aspects of April's life (family, school, friends, and other activities).

Professional assessment

Jenny had April go over the events of the last competition when she had lost contact with the pack. Jenny asked April to focus on three aspects of the race: (i) what she was thinking from start to finish, (ii) what her emotions were throughout the run, and (iii) what she did running-wise (overt behavior) in terms of strategies such as when she surged and when she drafted. April's thinking at the start, and throughout most of the race, contained a lot of "nots," such as "I am not going to lose contact at the end," "I am not going to draft when I could surge," and "I am not going to come in lower than third." Instructions about what *not to do* are usually unhelpful and often counterproductive. They leave images of failure in the mind with red lines through them. They do not instruct positively about what *to do*.

April's dominant emotion throughout the race was anxiety manifesting somatically with nausea and generalized muscle tension along with images of losing contact with the pack. Her race strategy went according to plan until the final two laps where her old patterns emerged, her self-talk went in the extremely negative direction and her anxiety rose substantially. Jenny asked for any other memories about the race. April mentioned that her dad was there on the far side of the track and would yell "Go! Go! Go!" each time she passed by, but she stated her problems happened at the ends of races whether her dad was at the competition or not.

Interventions

Jenny and April developed a plan for a two-pronged approach for her racing behavior. They began working on relaxation techniques aimed at reducing her generalized muscle tension. April started learning progressive muscle relaxation, which she would practice at home most days of the week, along with brief relaxation techniques she would use in practice and at competitions (e.g., body scans, diaphragmatic breathing). April and Jenny also began to catalog April's negative thinking patterns. They worked on identifying, and then stopping, negative thoughts (e.g., "I'm losing contact"), replacing them with positive affirmations (e.g., "Stay with them. Surge!").

April felt that she was getting a handle on her tension and negative thinking, and she used the relaxation and cognitive exercises everyday at practice and at home. Unfortunately, the somatic and cognitive training were not effective when it came to competition. In her next race, April performed just as she had done in the past, lost contact with the pack, and fell behind in the last two laps. April was disappointed, but Jenny explained that sometimes it takes awhile (and a lot of practice) to get new patterns of thinking and feeling into the "system." New ways of behaving and thinking are not stable at first and can be overwhelmed by the long-practiced "default" patterns that are solid features in the athlete's world. April continued to work hard on her mental skills, hoping they would kick in on her next competition.

Jenny thought that maybe there was something else going on for April. Jenny attended the next competition and had a brief chat with April before her race. It was a "home" competition, so Jenny asked April if her father was there. April said that he was the man in the red jacket on the far side of the track. Just before the race Jenny moved over to the far side about 10 m from where April's dad stood. During the race, April's dad was encouraging with shouts of "Go! Go! Go!" With two and a half laps to go, April was at the back of the pack, and she looked anxious. When she ran by, Jenny heard her dad yell "Don't lose contact again," and by the time she came around again she was about 12 m behind the pack. Her dad then yelled "Give it up and go home. You've lost it again."

Re-intervention

In their next session, Jenny described to April what she had observed during the last competition, and April began to cry. She had never cried in front of Jenny before, and so she became embarrassed and apologetic saying, "Sorry, I am such a baby," and the tears still flowed. Jenny felt she had some idea of where those tears came from (i.e., wanting love from a caring, supportive, but often psychologically abusive parent; wanting to please him, and repeated failures to do so). Jenny remembered something she had learned from reading her counseling education and training. She waited awhile in silence and then said, "April, I don't see you as a baby. I see you as a young woman who has kept a lot of pain inside for a long time. Maybe, the tears are telling us something important. If those tears had a voice, what would they tell us?"

Then a story of how much her dad had been so caring and gave her so much attention when she was young, how her success as a junior was the center of family pride, how her dad always wanted a son, how she moved from number 1 in the State as a secondary school runner to just another runner on her university team, and how disappointed her dad had been. Her

CASE STUDY (Continued)

love for her dad and wanting his approval and attention prevented her from telling Jenny the whole story early in their relationship. And herein lies the problem of sport psychology service delivery. All the relaxation and self-talk in the world may not have any salubrious effect if there is a much deeper and painful problem that is feeding the anxiety and negative self-talk. If those more subterranean problems are not unearthed, then the CBT interventions will be like band-aids placed over a deep wound. They may help stop or slow the bleeding, but they won't help the wound heal properly.

Jenny and April then spent several sessions talking about her relationship with her father. In many ways, he sounded like a loving and caring father, but when it came to her racing, he would become abusive. April told Jenny about her paternal grandfather and how he often belittled her father in front of his grandchildren about not providing for them well enough, not getting them into better schools, and so forth. Coaches coach as they were coached. Parents parent as they were parented. April's dad tried hard not to be like his psychologically abusive father, and for the most part he was successful, but when it came to high stress times (e.g., April's racing), he reverted back to patterns he learned early in his life.

About a week before her next race, Jenny met with April to discuss the upcoming competition. After going over her relaxation and self-talk, April fell silent, and looked a bit perplexed and sad. Jenny kept quiet, and eventually April said, "I know why my dad is the way he is, but I keep hearing, 'You've lost it. Go home!' in my head, and I just can't talk to him about it. Could you talk to him? I could tell him that my shrink would like to let him know what we are doing to prepare for the next race. Could you please do that for me?"

Outcome

Jenny had a long chat with April's father. He impressed her as a concerned parent who wanted to do the best for his child. She helped coach him in how to encourage her throughout the whole race. He seemed receptive, and they decided that they would stand together on the far side of the track while April raced. During the race April stayed with the pack, but when she went by Jenny and her dad with two and a half laps to go she was about 4 m behind the pack. As coached by Jenny, her dad yelled "You're doing fine sweetheart. You stay with them." At one and a half laps her father said "You're still there; You'll catch 'em!" And with one half of a lap to go the pack had strung out quite a bit, but April was in eigth place. At this point her dad yelled, "Go! Go! Go!" April passed three runners in the last 200 m and finished fourth. Lots of happiness and hugs all around.

April's issue, as first presented, was probably not the central one. In April's case (as in many others) there was an "issue behind the issue." It was only when Jenny got to the source of the issue behind the issue, and addressed it, that progress was made. The case of April and Jenny illustrates the potential multiple layers that may exist in sport psychology services, assessment, treatment, and outcome.

References

Sachs, M.L., Burke, K.L., Loughren, E.A. (2007) *Directory of Graduate Programs in Applied Sport Psychology*, 8th Edn. Fitness Information Technology, Morgantown, WVA.

Van Raalte, J.L., Andersen, M.B. (2007) When sport psychology consulting becomes a means to an end(ing): roles and agendas when helping athletes leave their sports. *The Sport Psychologist* **21**, 227–242.

Further reading

Andersen, M.B. (ed.) (2000) *Doing Sport Psychology*. Human Kinetics, Champaign, IL.

Andersen, M.B. (ed.) (2005) *Sport Psychology in Practice*. Human Kinetics, Champaign, IL.

Petitpas, A.J., Giges, B., Danish, S.J. (1999) The sport psychologist–athlete relationship: implications for training. *The Sport Psychologist* **13**, 344–357.

Index